The Unseen Universe:
Of Mind and Matter

Daniel Weiss Miller, Ph.D.

The Unseen Universe: Of Mind and Matter

Beyond The Realm Publishing / September 1993

Original Edition

For information address:
Beyond The Realm Publishing
106 St. Marks Ave.
Brooklyn, N.Y. 11217

Library of Congress Cataloging-in-Publication Data

ISBN 0-9638055-0-9

Library of Congress card catalogue number
93-73063

PRINTED IN THE UNITED STATES OF AMERICA

Dedicated to:

Jean Louis Cattaui, who spent his whole life as a New Age physicist before it ever began, and committed suicide despairing of ever reaching a sensitive, interested, aware public.

Table of Contents

Part I
Dynamics in the Quontic System

Chapter 1. Lost in the Fifth Dimension

Chapter 2. Consciousness: Defining Problems

Chapter 3. Models of Consciousness

Chapter 4. The Body-Mind at Work

Chapter 5. The Quontic System: Transmutations

Chapter 6. Consciousness Square
On Skyros

Part II
Quantum Physics: The Holes Within the Wholes

Chapter 7. Quantum Physical Reality

Chapter 8. The Purple Cow Dilemma

Chapter 9. Dimensions of Time and Memory: Travelling the Q-Loop

Chapter 10. Many Worlds — Many Times

Chapter 11. Regression in Brazil

Part III

How to Receive Messages from the Future Before They Are Sent

Chapter 12. Symmetry and Its Breaking, or, Is Dr. Weinberg Listening?

Chapter 13. Scalar Waves and Further Dynamics in the Quontic Loop

Chapter 14. Non-Linear Light Waves: Photonics

Chapter 15. Complementarism — Particle and Wave Revisited: Healing the Splits

Table of Figures

Introduction and Overview

The Beginning: Immersion in Experience

This book developed over many years, gestation occurring in the course of psychotherapy sessions with my clients and during personal and transpersonal experiences for which I had no rational explanations. During sessions I found the problems and transformation of many people holding hands while their unconscious awareness unfolded. Concepts emerged and whetted my excitement during long immersions in research reports in journals and books about everything I could lay my hands on in the biological sciences, physics and metaphysics, evolving into patterns that rubbed against my feet like a friendly cat. These patterns slowly grew into an integration of relationships that needed a name and the unifying name developed into Quontic Psychology. When I found a lack of words to describe what I meant I searched in the dictionary and if I couldn't find it there I coined a word, such as "quontic".

When people asked what "quontic" meant I would try to be brief by saying that it's about psychology of consciousness, science and metaphysics, but that always seemed inadequate. I'd prefer to say something like, "Quontic Psychology is a system which examines scientific, psychological and metaphysical aspects of information in order to discover interrelationships among them which will organize the psychodynamics of matter and mind into an integrated science", but I usually didn't have the time or the presence of mind for such an academic presentation.

It is obviously an enormous project, too much for one book. When people, with justified disbelief, asked me how long ago I began this book I jokingly replied about 700 years ago. After awhile I thought that it could have begun about 7000 years ago, if I included what I knew about my past lives. All things considered, the actual physical writing of it began with a Ph.D. thesis, in which I was skillfully guided by Stanley Krippner, in this life, and that only began about fifteen years ago. The last page here, I think, is simply an interruption.

Succinctly, this book is the product of a process of searching for an understanding which can bring together the variety of daily and non-ordinary experiences in which we live. The personal paranormal part of the search came to me involutarily in the midst of a psychotherapy session when a door opened to a past life experience. Although I'd known about and even participated voluntarily and involuntarily in psychic events prior to that, my commitment didn't become serious until the spontaneous regression to a past life happened.

In that sense, this book is additionally a history of my search for some way to understand the confusing contradictions of just being alive. I found that the paranormal experiences that I explored ultimately gave me an expanded focus on the events in my daily life and enriched my personal sense of involvement immensely. It also expanded my command of techniques as a psychologist after exploration and training with Roger Woolger (Woolger 1985). I was able to introduce past life regression into Organic Process Therapy. OPT was a process based on Gestalt (Perls 1969) and Primal (Janov 1970) techniques mainly until I included past lives. Training, to me, means immersing yourself in the therapy process as a patient to find out what it does for you before introducing it in your own practice. This intensive experiential work was what helped lead me further into paranormal experiences. My Ph.D. degree came later in life, from Greenwich University, where I am now an Adjunct Professor.

The Field of Non-Linear Research

Everyday life offers only one dimension of the total experience of existence, science offers only another, psychology just another and spiritual and paranormal belief systems yet another, and none of these cohere particularly well. Within each of these systems we have further fragmented our lives by focussing with equal fervor on special parts calling for experts such as specialists in Medicine, in the Sciences, in Religion, in Psychotherapy, etc. Science fragments itself by proliferating specialties and subspecialties, dividing its information into theories in basic chemistry, physics, biology, paleontology, archeology, etc., after which it divides and fragments mitotically into subspecialties. Then there are the prolific supermarket-shelf psychotherapies which offer instant cures in attractive packages to promise the best of all possible worlds. In the paranormal picture there are persons who appear to have specialized capabilities in avoiding reality with many eager converts ready to flee to the latest constellation of stars, led into an enchanted future by their favorite pied piper. It is much easier to go there than to return. For more patient searchers for understanding and self-development, this book will have a rich meaning.

Against all the best intentions, fragmentation in the fields of knowledge as well as daily life is inevitable. It cannot be totally deplored since it is intrinsic to the limited and specialized capacities for skilled absorption and comphrehension built into human functioning. Computers seem to have a better spread in this regard.

Despite the cynicism I've expressed, I know there are sincere and capable practitioners whose knowledge has depth enough to guide armchair astronauts into truly significant experiences (witness my own list of gurus and groups at the end of this introduction). Such experiences should stretch the limits and the borders of what a mind can include about a lifetime of past and potentially fascinating future events and experiences.

Finally, for me, exploration and discovery demands the meaningful assimilation of new information to see how it can make sense, particularly when it includes polar opposite subject matters such as the research found in scientific and paranormal journals. It is not a matter of right and wrong;

it is a matter of how to include all the sensible varieties of irreligious experience. A structure with which to do this is offered in Chapter 1, in the section on FOCUS.

This search for meaning to integrate what can and can't be seen has taken me, at times unwillingly kicking and screaming, (I still do Primal Therapy) into the paranormal dimension very actively. The most conscious phase of this search began about 1970 when I inadvertently stumbled into my first past life experience following a very intensive rebirthing therapy session. It opened up the door to an interest in physics, which surprised me since I had no prior proclivity in that direction. I was suddenly faced with the fact that my work as a psychologist had led me into strange, unfamiliar, contradictory territory by pulling me into both the parapsychological-metaphysical-spiritual dimension and the physical sciences simultaneously. There are no two more incompatible dimensions of existence because parapsychology is elusive to testing "in the real world" and the other, science, is supposedly a proven guide to reality (even when it is continually acknowledging errors and altering its conclusions through its experimental procedures.)

As time, experience and study progressed, the contradictions and the validity of both dimensions became more apparent. It lead to my joining both the American Society for Psychical Research and the New York Academy of Sciences, with dedication to the valid purposes of each. Their conflicts and splits, like a divorced couple who could be enthralled with each other if they could forget their quarrels, were in need of healing through a unifying paradigm. I concluded that each understands significant but different aspects of the way the world works. Their opposition reflects our inner fragmentation, as well as thralldom to positions taken over by egoism and personal gain, which we shall also investigate in these pages.

The issue of a need for a unifying paradigm has become a broader, more dangerous issue. It includes personal and social well-being, the mental and physical health of the individual, of the society, and of the planet itself. There is greater awareness than ever that we lead fragmented lives, split off from ourselves, from each other, from our earth, air and water. Splitting ourselves off emotionally from our spiritual and social selves is reflected in the indifference of economic man freely polluting and vandalizing his environment, smoking and eating himself to death without self-concern or awareness, not caring that one man's smoke is another man's cancer. However, ignorance is not bliss. Our unbalanced lives are also reflected in the destroyed homeostasis of the planet. Our continued survival needs a paradigm that will unify us internally, with each other and with the wonderfully inexplicable environment on which we depend for our fragile lives.

To try for a reintegration of all that diversity is undoubtedly an ambitious undertaking, but it is made easier with the concepts of FOCUS and homeostasis. Homeostasis is presented in various chapters as a basic, unifying principle which permeates every level of existence and serves as a governor of daily events from the level of the atom to the relationships of the planets. Not least of all, homeostasis guides the relationships of the internal mechanisms of the physiological and psychological self in the human organism. There will be a great deal of effort expended in this book describing how homeostasis is clearly a vital part of a psychophysiological feedback system impacting consciousness. It is taken up extensively in Chapter 4, "The Bodymind at Work".

The centrality of homeostasis in this process will be elaborated to show how it is linked to survival and memory. Although homeostasis is a powerful directive with a give and take interacting with feedback systems within the organism, it can also be thrown off course and prevented from functioning adequately. "Dehomeosis", one of several words I've coined to fill up a conceptual gap, is the result of dysfunctional behavior which destroys homeostasis. It seems that dysfunctional behavior has become the norm these days and the dehomeotic state is being fostered by government, medicine and even science. Physical and psychological illness are barometric gauges of the homeostatic state from the person's feedback system regarding internal relationships. Dehomeosis is reflected, on a larger scale, in the increasing illness of our planet, as well as our selves.

The Search for Uncertainty

We hold onto Reality as hard as possible by being economic, practical and scientific, with extraordinarily frustrating results. Nevertheless it is very hard to let go of the economic, scientific, medical approach to reality. That would create an anxiety because once we stray too far from the path into paranormal and spiritual dimensions the way becomes unclear, strewn with hazardous rubble. Reality as we have known it loses its boundaries, its framework starts to bend and, like gravity, the shape of it becomes hard to see. Is it possible to live with this kind of uncertainty?

Is it possible to say that you don't know all the particulars, that the way into the picture and the way through it is not clear? The psychic astronaut can be conflictually lead by intuitive forces into worlds which are experientially felt as known but not sponsored by any of the usual physical senses. Ultimately, you may find yourself traveling along an unseen way into an unseen universe. Then, if you want to continue, all you can do is trust yourself and the forces that guide you because the usual signposts are gone. Chapters 6 and 11 are devoted to Organic Process Therapy sessions at Skyros Center, Greece and Pax Center in Sao Paolo, Brazil. During workshops, participants followed the signposts along the unseen way and found healing.

In panic, we keep running back to the practical, economic and scientific explanations, but they no longer satisfy. Indeed scientists too have lost their signposts and, as in quantum physics, which we take up in Chapter 7, they have had to make Uncertainty into a basic principle of quantum physical life. A reevaluation of what was only possible became necessary to make uncertainty certain.

I selectively took from what seemed to me the most significant fields of research in science, psychology and metaphysics and combined them without regard for provability, content that this too was in the range of what's "only possible". Thus, the "irrational" universe of quontic psychology in Chapter 5 does not depend on scientific proof for the verification of its hypotheses even though many of its sources are scientific. At the present time, allowing the unknown to present itself creatively is the only way to integrate the most vital aspects of all the known and intuited data.

Clearly, the purpose of this book is not to produce another scientific theory, even though it relies a lot upon science for many of its ideas, but to make comprehensible to myself and hopefully therefore to others how it is possible to live with experiences providing information whose sources and interpretations appear hopelessly opposed to conventional and scientific descriptions of reality. This ultimately impinges on the question of what is reality, how to recognize delusional processes, and the issue of what constitutes sanity, including my own, at times. And why not? If a psychologist can't question his own sanity, or the givens in his reality, then he has no right to ask other people to question theirs. In other words, in taking risks, my tolerance for swings in the way I deal with reality gets stretched to the limit sometimes and appears to threaten my personal homeostasis. However, with practice, one becomes resilient, allows for changes and maintains one's confidence in a core of adequate and competent functioning. It becomes comforting to realize one doesn't lose the sense of reality one has had for forty, fifty or sixty years by allowing it to expand while exploring paranormal experiences. With flexibility, the either-or of sane or insane becomes changed and merges into the continuum.

An Overview of All That Is and Is Not

A brief preview of *The Unseen Universe: Of Mind and Matter*, such as this, has to be based on its purpose - closing the gap between the operations of mind and matter. Part II is a review of contemporary physics theory and continues the attempt to unify "rational" with "irrational" science. Part III looks at ways that science has already, albeit unwittingly, conceptually closed the gap.

Central to all this is the concept of homeostasis and its expression in Quontic Psychology. Homeostasis will be briefly described here and fully explained in a later chapter. Homeostasis is treated somewhat unconventionally insofar as it is not viewed as a static point of things in balance but as participating in a fairly wide range of behaviors and activities—not as the fulcrum of a see-saw but as the range of movement of the see-saw. This is portrayed in Figure 1., *Homeostasis*, showing homeostasis can operate like a seesaw effectively within a certain range as long as it isn't compelled by the mechanism or the organism to get stuck somewhere by having equal weights on each end or by becoming so overweighted on one end it becomes immobilized. Homeostasis functions effectively only within the role of creator, mover and limiter maintaining interactive activities.

At the higher functioning level is the Homeostatic Principle, which is responsible, like a thermostat, for regulating the general universe, operating by keeping systems within their effective range of function as best it can. But it is not always successful. People, organisms with consciousness, themselves subject to the operation of the principle, have become sophisticated at defeating it, to their own ultimate self-destruction. Consciousness, with the best of intentions, is not always its own savior.

Consequently there is mental and physical illness, war, homocides and suicides, drug addiction and all the other behaviors that indicate the functions of the "thermostat" are losing the ability to contain the limits of behavior within the homeostatic range. People take corrective measures such as

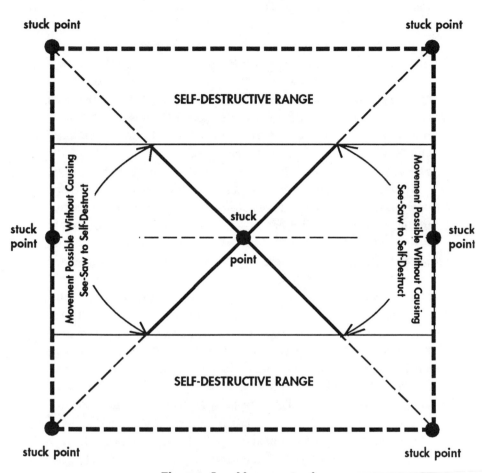

Figure 1. Homeostasis,

showing homeostasis can operate like a seesaw effectively within a certain range as long as it isn't compelled by the mechanism or the organism to get stuck.

seeing psychotherapists, doctors, priests, finding new jobs and new lovers and unfortunately take drugs in an attempt to restore homeostasis. Defeat the homeostatic mechanisms in both your psychophysiology and the environment in which you live and you ultimately destroy yourself and your environment.

What Humans Do to Destroy It

It is so commonplace and free that we take it for granted, like air and water. But if we look at it more closely, it is a master program whose application is everywhere and crucial to everything. Homeostasis is the result of parts working in relation to each other providing feedback through connecting networks of transmission lines, pipes or organs which keep the parts and the system informed and nourished with needed supplies.

In people, organ systems feed into consciousness which has memories about experiences of how both to operate homeostatically and how it was, or fears how it would be, to lose the homeostatic baseline. Consciousness is considered to be, in the quontic system, an evolved, large-scale organizer for the homeostatic principle.

Maintainance of homeostasis for life is a necessity, not a luxury. Why and how then do we defeat it? We destroy it out of a lack of awareness of its importance. People, like forestland and plant life, can take a certain amount of abuse until they break down into illness which then demands strong, effective treatment to restore it to its homeostatic range, or it will die. Like its people, the earth has become sick through defeat of its natural homeostatic mechanisms.

One of the ways we manifest lack of awareness is through socially supported attitudes which fragment everything into bits and pieces instead of seeing the network of interactions necessary to keep a system whole and healthy. This shortage of awareness occurred in industry, and has become particularly acute in the medical establishment which is now consequently in a state of crisis.

True, there is a certain amount of inevitability in breaking things down into smaller manageable parts when the system is very large. Though it becomes more manageable, breaking a part down for analysis also results in treating that part as if it were isolated, external to the system. However, the part that is treated and changed needs to have these changes made in such a way that they are related functionally to the rest of the system so that a healthy homeostasis can reform itself. Lacking awareness, it comes as a surprise to people on medication that they can suffer harmful side-effects from taking a drug intended to make them healthy - meant to restore the organismic balance and not to destroy it further.

The problem is generic to our Western scientific attitudes which have created polarities of function such as subjective and objective instead of seeing differences in terms of continuities, such as the yin and yang of Eastern philosophy. We deal in Mind vs Matter, Right vs Wrong, Good vs Evil, Material vs Spiritual, People vs Nature and in warfare with a nation fixated in one category of politics against a nation fixated in another political category. We haven't developed an appreciation of the Complementariness in physical and psychological events, which the great physicist Niels Bohr pointed out and is further described in Chapter 14.

Mind vs matter fragmentation is depicted in the following diagram, Figure 2., *Synchronistic Perception in a Fragmented State*, showing perception and homeostasis fragmented by blocks in the lower half as well as by the diameter-barrier dividing the circle into two halves.

The lower half represents mundane reality, the three-dimensional, scientific, material aspect of life with fragmentation due to blocks and barriers separating what would otherwise be connected. The upper half represents spiritual reality, the metaphysical, paranormal, or as we shall call it, the fifth-dimensional aspect of the whole. Neither section alone deals with the entire reality which we shall call Unifunctional - appreciating the essentially integrated connections among the mental and physical parts that make up the whole Gestalt which finally is larger than the sum of the parts in the unifunctional system. The outcome of dealing with reality unifunctionally is the preservation of homeostasis, which moves in continuity around the circle.

Behind and underneath fragmentation lies a paradox. Dividing large matters up helps to deal with problems of daily life whether through science, economics, technology, or even in interpersonal relationships with greater ease than at-

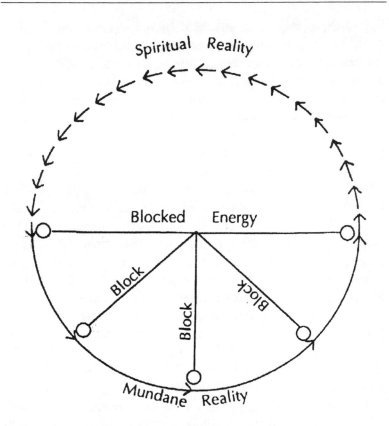

Figure 2.
Synchronistic Perception in a
Fragmented State,

showing perception and homeostasis fragmented by blocks
in the lower half as well as by the diameter-barrier dividing the circle.

tempting to deal with the unifunctional picture continually.
It may thereby, for the moment, temporarily enhance survival. On the other hand, the results remain fragmented -
incomplete and ultimately destructive, defeating homeostasis, and threatening survival.

However, there are certainly things that can be done to lessen the impact of fragmentation and increase homeostasis. One of these would be to create a FOCUS, that is, a Field of Complex Unifunctional Studies to integrate the external sources of knowledge about our world with the internal sources of knowledge about ourselves in the world described in Chapter 1, "The Fifth Dimension".

Survival Anxiety On Tap — As Below So Above

Figure 3., *Survival and Culture*, shows how basic survival anxiety kneads its way up through the individual, the family, society and into the culture.

A way that our culture has been affected by science was to divide knowledge into categories of objective, materialistic, scientific "rational" information and subjective, psychological, spiritual, metaphysical, "irrational" information. Being "objective" helps an investigator to believe he is getting a true grasp on reality and thus is able to cope with survival anxiety.

Survival anxiety is a very important motivating factor in many areas of activity. For instance people work and relate at jobs and with others whom they'd rather not need to have in their lives, or they remain tied within relationships which are mutually destructive. The problem of survival anxiety actually begins during pre-birth, in the womb, and is geometrically increased during the birth process (Miller 1977, 1978).

Psychotherapy shows that birth is where contact with the possibility of death is first known as a living human experience. Experiences at those times and in later infancy and childhood either aggravate or help soften the anxiety but it probably never disappears completely. Among the things that money can't buy should be added the elimination of survival anxiety. However, it may be modified and reduced with effective, aware psychotherapy and altered with a spiritual belief system. This is also a theme that runs throughout this book.

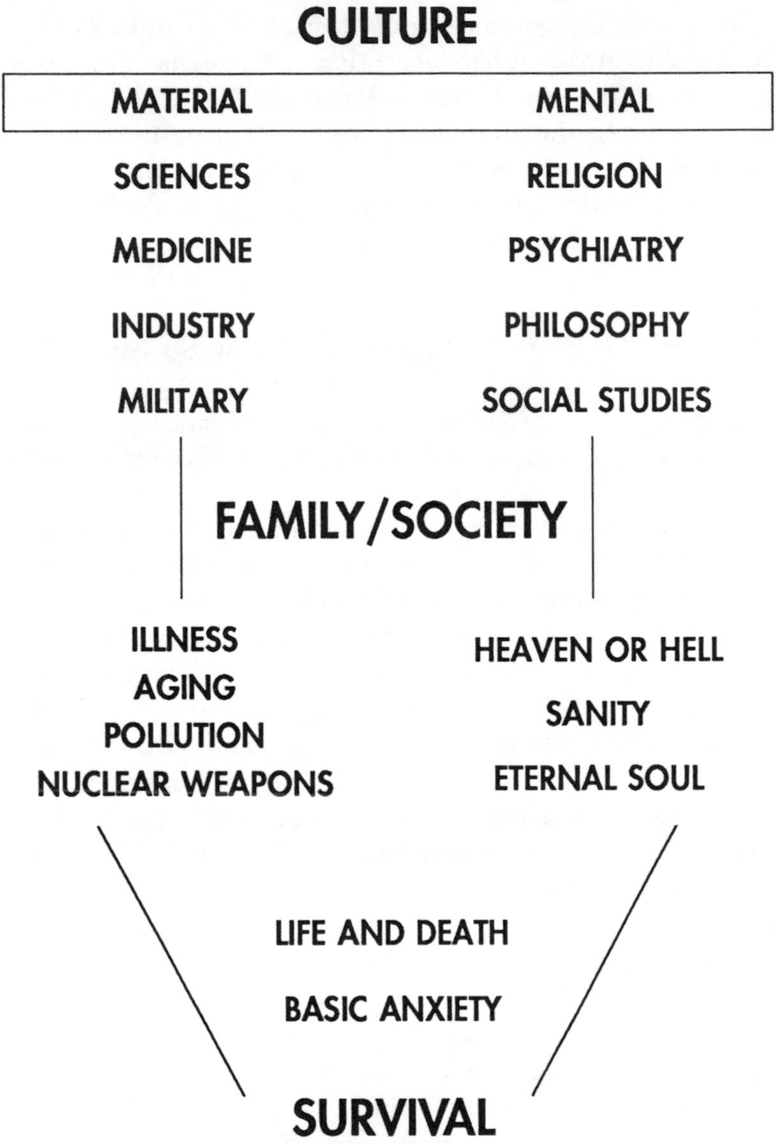

CULTURE

MATERIAL	MENTAL
SCIENCES	RELIGION
MEDICINE	PSYCHIATRY
INDUSTRY	PHILOSOPHY
MILITARY	SOCIAL STUDIES

FAMILY/SOCIETY

ILLNESS
AGING
POLLUTION
NUCLEAR WEAPONS

HEAVEN OR HELL
SANITY
ETERNAL SOUL

LIFE AND DEATH

BASIC ANXIETY

SURVIVAL

Figure 3.
Survival and Culture,

shows how basic survival anxiety kneads its way up
through the individual, the family, and society into the
culture.

On the next page is Figure 4., *How Survival Affects Consciousness*. Survival anxiety affects feelings and thoughts, mind and body, attitudes toward spirit and matter, influencing and creating memories regarding homeostasis via a feedback system.

The feedback system exchanges information within different levels of memory to bring awareness to consciousness. However, the resulting information bank has to first negotiate its way through ego defenses which determine whether or not it can pass into consciousness. Chapters 3, "Models of Consciousness" and 9, "Dimensions of Time and Memory" elaborate this topic.

Consciousness and Self

Consciousness functions as a screen to display thoughts, feelings, memories, body states and everything else below its level, after filtration by the ego defenses. Scientific neurobiology has contributed much to our current psychological understanding of how body states relate to memory, though many questions remain. The ego's trained effort to create a socially acceptable self-concept may have little to do with the real, organic, homeostatic version of the self-concept developed in the crucible of the unconscious from the impact of developmental personal experience. This will become related to psychological states which are conventionally labelled "normal or abnormal", or as we prefer to call them, stable, homeostatic or pseudohomeostatic, unstable or dehomeotic..

Case studies in Chapter 6 illustrate this distinction.

Definitions:
1. **Stable** - Regulated, tends toward rigidity
2. **Homeostatic** - Maximally effective movement
3. **Pseudohomeostatic** - Artificial facade, unreal "normal", compensated.
4. **Unstable** - Moves in and out of homestasis
5. **Dehomeotic** - Very little homeostasis left

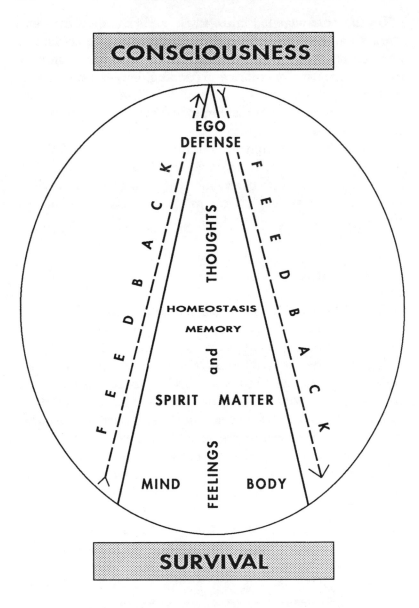

Figure 4.
How Survival Affects Consciousness

Survival anxiety affects feelings and thoughts, mind and body, attitudes toward spirit and matter, influencing and creating memories.

Sexual behavior, as an example, runs the gamut in the route from the homeostatic, unconscious, organic level of the body-mind, through ego-defended filtration where it may become pseudo-homeostatic or unstable in consciousness. Sexuality runs a course between Scylla and Charybdis, between its physiology and a variety of developmental memories and ego defenses, on the path to constructing a reality regarding sexual behavior dominated by a social self-concept (if it has not become so unstable as to become dehomeotic) which is what consciousness perceives and displays.

Generally, the further apart the organically real and the ego-dominated self-images, the greater the internal, physiological and social conflict, neurosis, and illness a person will experience. These dynamics relate closely to the status and the work of homeostasis which is also affected by the degree of survival anxiety that a person has to integrate from the beginning of his/her life through birth and subsequent experiences. These observations may be just as true of persons with cancer as those with a psychosis, though the outcome may have been directed through a different path in each case.

The end result of this process of intricately networked relationships, reflected in the contents of consciousness and health, is obviously drawn from a complex compilation from the warehouse of events, memories, and information related to homeostasis and survival in mundane third-dimensional and harmonic fifth-dimensional levels. Recent animal research reported in Chapter 4 indicates that dreams also may fundamentally be an invention of consciousness to aid in processing survival anxiety. All that is preparation for the quontic model.

Two major models of consciousness, a Western psychophysiological and an Eastern metaphysical model are compared in this book in Chapter 3. Their contributions also feed into quontic psychology.

QUONTIC PSYCHOLOGY

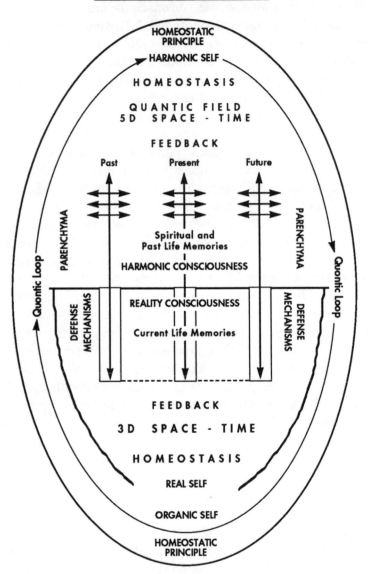

Figure 5.
The Egg of Consciousness in Quontic Psychology

The shell of it is homeostasis; crack that and the entire
system disintegrates.

Quontic Psychology

On the facing page, Figure 5., is *The Egg of Consciousness in Quontic Psychology.* The shell of it is homeostasis; crack that and the entire system disintegrates.

The organic self is the essential component of the person. It maintains psychophysiological connections within the body. With the real self, it is the interface between the physiological and psychological homeostatic aspects of consciousness.

From the organic self to consciousness, a feedback process of information exchange between internal psychophysiological, external environmental and meta-physical sources of stimulation feed each other with input. What follows then is the possibility of deriving a homeostasis within the person receiving input from oftentimes discrepant internal, external and harmonic data. Bringing such data into balance is an awesome challenge for the individual in his life (as well as for the writer of this book). However, the effort is essential. The totality of the system of relationships, paranormal as well as mundane, geared toward the survival of the organism through the operation of the Homeostatic Principle, is what I have called Quontic Psychology.

In Figure 5, the upper and lower halves are the fifth and third dimensions, respectively. They are connected through the quontic loop which is the channel for the network of relationships between fifth or "harmonic" and third or "reality" dimensions of spacetime. The barrier that separates them is the fourth dimension, which is the barrier of the speed of light, 186,000 miles per sec. All this will be extensively clarified in Chapter 5, which takes up the quontic psychological system in detail.

An Irrational Science

The Many Worlds Theory, the Holographic Theory and Group Symmetry Theory (Chapters 10 and 12) make vital contributions to "the science of the irrational". These are in the last third of the book which is somewhat more demanding in toleration of scientific expression in that it examines concepts in quantum physics and relativity to see what ideas can be derived that will satisfy the quontic psychological purpose of integrating science with the paranormal. Indeed, we will find there are large loopholes in scientific explanations of reality which tend to support the unifunctional way of looking at ourselves and at our universe. It seems that it is quite a valid notion to support the idea of a Field of Complex Unifunctional Studies, whose outgrowth is Quontic Psychology, as a sensitive and necessary way to integrate ourselves with the universe. We are affected by and in turn affect everything that goes on around us.

That the FOCUS approach extends in degree to the fabled butterfly which flaps its wings in China and causes a storm in Mexico, as goes the claim in chaos theory, is probably too weird to believe. But that CFC's released in New York and London would cause a hole over the Antartic that can cause cancer in unwary sunbathers and cause climactic changes all over the world would have sounded equally ridiculous just a few years ago. Minimally, that we have more of an impact and are impacted by our environment much more than we ever thought possible is a reasonably irrational statement.

As is so often the case, intuitive poets and philosophers have written in this vein for hundreds of years, "Ask not for whom the bell tolls, it tolls for thee." It is taking an ecological disaster to give the dimensions of the idea its formidable meaning. Therefore, Chapter 14 contains a Plan For The Twenty-First Century—not grandiose, perhaps not even impressive, but in some variation essential for returning psychological and physical homeostasis to the planet.

I do not, and this is important to keep in the foreground as one reads, hopefully, to the end of this book - I repeat, I do not offer final solutions because I do not believe that such things exist in reality. The process of engaging in the search and developing an integration that has room for doubt is the essence of this book, even when the ideas presented are neatly wrapped up in a scientific presentation. These scientifically wrapped ideas helped me to organize and to tell others about what I think I currently know, in other words, they have become a delicately held paradigm. I don't need to cling to them to resolve my issues about reality. I'm aware there are contradictions and multiple explanations for the same phenomena, but as I said, this is more like an exploration of what is only possible, a "thought experiment", rather than a final answer. To present one would be foolish because there is no final answer; there is just the evolutionary unfolding process between mind and matter.

The people who will probably find it easiest to read this book? Probably the college educated layman or student who threw away his interest in psychology, science and spiritual matters too early, to his regret, and wishes to make up for lost time. The person, young or old, educated or not, embarked on a search perhaps for truth, perhaps for interrelations of supposed truths, questioning everything skeptically in order to make up his own mind. The person wanting to process his own paranormal experiences in the light of another person's to see what new ideas can be gleaned, to charge his own beliefs. The person, sometimes a professional negative critic of the paranormal, sometimes a scientist, who has read all the other books of this type, fearful he might find one that will be scientifically valid and convincing, but fortunately for his peace of mind, never does. I trust that the majority of people who don't fit into any of these stereotypes will enjoy reading it as well.

No book could be written without numerous people who have, with or without intention, contributed substantially to its development. Professional groups which gave me the freedom to explore my ideas such as the International Metaphysical Conferences and Pax Center in Sao Paolo, Brazil, the Skyros Center directed by Dina Glouberman and Jannis Andricopolous in Greece, the Association for Past Life Research and Therapies and the International Primal Association and their clients and colleagues; not to mention those patients in my private practice, currently in Brooklyn, who sometimes unwittingly supported me by contributing their own experiences and lessons adapted to these pages. Certainly Dr.Stanley Krippner and Dr. Elizabeth Mintz who were stalwart friends and associates above and beyond the call of duty. The Emissary Foundation in Garden City, N.Y., a body of people committed to loving and creative awareness, and mutual support. I should not leave out Buddhist groups such as Sydda Yoga and Yeshe Nyingpo and their gurus, the late Muktananda succeeded by Guramay and the late Dudjom Rimpoche who was succeeded by his son Shenphen whose training sessions helped form my spiritual awareness. Regula Noetzli who, as literary agent, helped patiently and knowingly by guiding my writing into a better form, and unnamed but not forgotten friends whose consistent support and encouragement at various times helped bring it to completion. And finally, appreciation to my children, Larissa, David and Sarah (who did some of the diagrams) who still aren't sure what to make of a father who did workshops in Europe on his birthday, conducted therapy sessions that entered dangerous primal waters using unorthodox methods, and taught strange things that most other fathers ignored or scoffed at.

Finally, I must take complete responsibility for this book's contents since I had few opportunities to discuss these ideas with other psychologists, scientists or writers. Exceptions to that were avant garde journal editors like Harris Dienstfrey, of Advances, Bob Reiber of Social Distress and Homelessness, and Mickel Adzema of Primal Renaissance, who also published my articles. And bouquets as well to those who, even in small ways, opposed my ideas for I always thrive well on opposition.

July 20, 1993

Brooklyn, N.Y.

Part I

Dynamics
in the
Quontic System

Lost in the Fifth Dimension

Albert Einstein:

"Poor old Joffre can't make up his mind through which hole an electron will go if he fires it through a lead obstacle with a number of holes. An electron is indivisible, and therefore it must go through one hole only. But which hole? And the solution" — with a gust of Einstein laughter — "is really very simple: it goes through the fifth dimension."

from Einstein, the Life and Times
by R. W. Clark [1]

Looking at Scientific Method

What are we looking at when we deal with paranormal and metaphysical experience? The question is becoming more and more important because of the growing number of persons who are willing to consider psychic experience an actual fact of life. Scientists insist that such preoccupations are nonsensical products of irrational thinking. Investigators calling themselves "psicops" (psychic police) try to prove that psychic phenomena are a form of vaudeville magic that charlatans practice. People going through psychic experiences such as forseeing a future event sometimes think they are going crazy and reject it completely. Should we simply accept these negative ways of seeing psychic experience or pursue it despite the risks involved? Is there any way of integrating psychic experience with the realities of daily life and scientific explanations?

Society, with its increasing acceptance of "irrational" experiences, is ahead of science in understanding the nature of reality. Included in "irrational" experiences are paranormal phenomena such as ESP (non-sensory communication between two persons), clairvoyance (ability to foresee future events), psychokinesis (moving objects with mental, non-physical means), psychic healing (healing illness with mental or spiritual energy, without medical intervention), past life regression (the ability to relive a prior lifetime with full awareness of emotional and situational events) and channelling (the ability to receive messages from the spirit world of etheric entities).

However, these are clearly non-traditional, unconventional, alternative sources of information. Accepting such experiences means, for the average person who has not experienced anything like it before, having access to mental powers and capabilities that only shamans, witches and priests were considered heir to at one time. It often creates a good deal of conflict in terms of the self-concept's long-standing preconceptions about the natural borders and limitations of reality. If he/she ("he" includes "she" hereafter) accepts this ability as real, what will he be able to do that he can't do now - and should he be the one to have the ability? If he enters into a past life is it real or just the imagination playing tricks on him? Or is he actually going crazy? Is there anybody he can tell and not be considered crazy?

Scientists ought to be more sophisticated about such matters, but many of them are not. They have as many doubts, anxieties and fears about paranormal phenomena as non-scientists, and in some cases, more. In additon to those personal anxieties, their reputations for accuracy and being right are at stake. They need proof that they have control over the correct, scientific representation of reality because that is how their work status is defined.

Science provides a special, careful way of altering the basic concepts of reality. The scientific method provides experimentation, repetition of the experiment by others and mathematization of results as sine qua non for research before any one may alter any notions about reality. Theories are only as reliable as experimentation can prove them to be. It is such a careful process that those who break the rules like Freud and Pasteur had difficulty being accepted at first, and psychology is still not considered a "real" science because its findings are sometimes impossible to measure and replicate and therefore very hard to control and prove. Even Einstein's theories of relativity were rejected for almost fifteen years because there was no proof. At first, it was just theory.

Prior to relativity, in 1905 Einstein had demonstrated and theoretically proved the existence of molecules which, at that time, were invisible to the human eye. He wrote of those physicists who rejected his theories:

> "The antipathy of these scholars towards atomistic theory can indubitably be traced back to their positivistic philosophical attitude. This is an interesting example of the fact that even scholars of audacious spirit and fine instinct can be obstructed in the interpretation of facts by philosophical prejudices. The prejudice-which has by no means died out in the meantime-consists in the faith that facts by themselves can and should yield scientific knowledge without free conceptual construction." [2]

"Free conceptual construction" is now called ad hoc theory and intuition. A scientific model which can incorporate psychic experience and paranormal experimentation is called for.

**The Field of Complex Unifunctional Studies:
FOCUS**

"A sand castle is thermodynamically
deeper than a sand dune, because the conscious
act of a child's packing wet sand into a hard mass
and then sculpting it into the facsimile of a
turreted medieval fortress involves more information than do the geological and meteorological
forces that conspire to make dunes. For one
thing, when measuring the breadth and thermo-
dynamic depth of the sand castle one must account not only for the natural processes that
result in a sandy beach, but also for the evolutionary processes that created the child....In practice,
of course, there are serious stumbling blocks,
since no one has the slightest idea what, say, the
breadth of a child might be. But that is no
objection to the principle behind the
definition....The study of complexity aims at understanding not only the origins of life but also
the possibilities for its future evolution." (Lloyd
1990 P.44 [3])

Though in their spiritual essence they may be simple, in
their manifestation to us the manifold patterns of nature are
complex. The essence of nature, expressed in its pristine
unitary form as a spiritual force is the way it is comprehended
in metaphysics whereas the comprehension of the mundane,
material, scientific universe finds itself enmeshed in a complex, fragmented, often confusing and unyielding form.
Attempting to understand nature's complexity through science has led us into the fracturing expressed in the multitude
of splits in scientific disciplines and their sub-disciplines.
The whole that we know exists through spiritual and metaphysical experience becomes lost in the proliferation of practical and scientific parts. It is very difficult to distill all this
fragmentation down to return nature to its wholeness.

Nevertheless, there has been enormous benefit conferred upon our way of life by the discoveries of scientific research. How can we keep the benefits of both approaches?

If we wish to see nature differently, more primally, integrated as more than the sum of its self-evident parts, yet without discarding the information laboriously gathered by scientists over several hundred years, we need another approach than the standard one offered by science. An alternative research method is taken if, while appreciating the unity and simplicity inherent in complexity, we look for explanations which use and integrate as much information from every branch of science as is possible to find out how we can distill their findings into fundamental principles which includes data from consciousness and paranormal concepts. This approach enables us to see patterns which overlap, coincide, merge and emerge into new relationships, similar to that which occurs when turning a kaleidoscope. We may see many alternative patterns arising from the same data, not just one pattern. What we can achieve through a reformulation and synthesis of data is, if not a statement of the essence, at least a position that represents a reflected image of the essence through observing its parts in interaction.

The way bacteria, people, and snowflakes behave depends very much on what is going on around them as well as what potentials arise from their internal structures. Structures have been evolutionarily engaged through the homeostatic, feedback process to perform certain jobs under certain conditions in nature. However, variability is also intrinsic to nature, therefore conditions change and stresses that create changes in structures which are responsive and flexible are essential to the continuing survival of all organic and inorganic matter. Taking knowledge from a variety of sources and disciplines in order to focus how those interactions occur and understanding their effects is also critical for scientific investigation.

Acknowledging complexity means finding as much information as possible from as many sources as possible, ideally.

However, with the enormous assistance provided by the computerization of information, the amount available is voluminously overwhelming. Therefore a careful selection of kinds and sources of data must be made.

Viewing science from the standpoint of complexity is not a new idea. As early as 1981 Fritjof Capra, interviewed by Renee Weber, envisioned an integration of scientific studies based on dynamic interactions and relationships between systems in very different scientific fields, creating a new paradigm for scientific research. He stated:

> "I have come to believe that in the future we will apply a network of models, and we will use different languages to describe different phenomena at different levels. We will not worry any longer whether we are doing biology or psychology or physics or anthropology or whatever; we won't be worried about these classifications." (Wilbur 1982 [4])

Heinz Pagels, the former Executive Director of the New York Academy of Sciences and a prominent physicist, in an issue of Science Focus stated the case clearly in a letter titled "Complexity, A New Synthesis of the Sciences".

> "...New ideas are now appearing in the way the sciences are ordered and divided. The physicist, Murray Gell-Mann, caught the spirit of this change in his remarks in 1984 to participants in the Santa Fe Institute, a new center for the study of complexity....
> "This movement has...to do with...the realization by specialized researchers that their scientific problems overlap those of investigators in disparate fields. People investigating neural nets, parallel processors, the immune response, the economic system, pattern recognition, the evolutionary system, autocatalytic reactions...

are discovering the common ground for understanding all these problems. It may herald a new synthesis of knowledge based on the idea of complexity....

"A new world view is laboring to be born as scientists move to examine the vast realm of complex systems. The knowledge derived from this will have a transforming effect on the way society is organized and how it uses information and technology....Advanced societies must begin now to accept the challenge of this new frontier in science." (Pagels 1987 [5])

Karl Pribram, a neuropsychologist, depicts a more narrow, relevant aspect of the problem succinctly when he says:

"...Modern physicists and modern perceptual psychologists have converged onto a set of issues that neither can solve alone. If the psychologist is interested in the nature of the conditions which produce the world of appearances, he must attend to the inquiries of the physicist. If the physicist is to understand the observations which he is attempting to systematize, he must learn something of the nature of the psychological process of making observations." (Wilber 1982 [6])

Even prior to this, in 1964, Nobel Prize winning physicist Richard P. Feynman gave a series of lectures at Cornell in which he foresaw the necessity of integrating a large variety of scientific theories. In one lecture, he stated:

"Which end is nearer to God; if I may use a religious metaphor. Beauty and hope, or the fundamental laws? I think that the right way, of course, is to say that what we have to look at is the whole structural interconnection of the thing;

and that all the sciences, and not just the sciences
but all the efforts of intellectual kinds, are an
endeavor to see the connections of the hierar-
chies, to connect beauty and history, to connect
history to man's psychology, man's psychology to
the working of the brain, the brain to the neural
impulse, the neural impulse to the chemistry,
and so forth, up and down, both ways....
"And I do not think either end is nearer to God. To
stand at either end, and to walk off that end of the
pier only, hoping that out in that direction is the
complete understanding, is a mistake. And to
stand with evil and beauty and hope, or to stand
with the fundamental laws, hoping that way to
get a deep understanding of the whole world,
with that aspect alone, is a mistake. It is not
sensible for the ones who specialize at one end,
and the ones who specialize at the other end, to
have such disregard for each other...."
(Feynman 1990 [7])

This extraordinary statement from a renowned physicist
sounds like a trumpet call for the integration of all the studies
of mankind including psychology and parapsychology. However, this is not the way it actually is. Later on, in another
lecture when he must have forgotten what he said in this one,
he denigrates psychology and parapsychological studies,
returns to the traditional scientific model and rejects any
claims they might have to scientific status for the commonplace reasons we have already mentioned and will expand
upon later.

Nevertheless, when scientists become irrational, there is
a recognized need for the inclusion of all disciplines into a
paradigm of some kind. Currently, many recent publications
on the relationship between quantum physics, psychology
and spirituality have been presented to the public. Concepts
are needed that can allow them to be integrated. Paranormal
research also suffers because it lacks a model that includes

both physical science as well as psychical and spiritual knowledge.

The currently official "Science of Complexity", despite Pagels' generous statements about joining the different scientific fields of study into one science, also excludes psychological and paranormal studies, that is to say, it omits the experiential part of being human. Therefore the approach which does include these two pariahs into science needs another name. It might be more aptly called, "The Field of Complex Unifunctional Studies", or FOCUS, to distinguish it from the aborted science of complexity.

It is important to affirm the validity of examining paranormal experience from both scientific and psychological points of view. Much has already been learned about human functioning from paranormal research, with an enormous body of work from the esoteric to the experimental, that has already convinced many of its validity. As a psychologist conducting a therapy practice which includes past life regression, I am inclined to pay special attention to the way in which all healing processes, including past lives and psychic healing, are derived from explanations seen through FOCUS. It's outcome is Quontic Psychology which attempts to fill out a contribution to the elusive picture drawn by science, esoteric religion and psychology, whose combined long-range vision is to portray the nature and place of humanity in the universe.

To accomplish this it becomes important for the reader to learn something about quantum physics and relativity, the psychology of memory and consciousness, something about the way the nervous system functions, and to review evolutionary processes or else we will never understand the whole picture of the human being experiencing something as extraordinary as this life, a past life, nor any other normal or paranormal event. Such is the diagram of Figure 6 on the next page. FOCUS indicates the complexity of scientific researches that have gone into the development of Quontic Psychology.

Each of the sides of the cube in Figure 6 represents a particular field of study. At the center is included the human

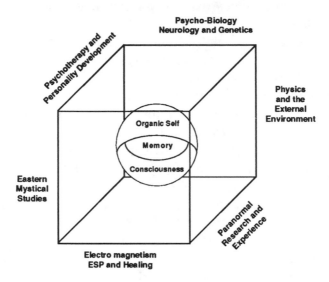

Figure 6.
Complexity in Quontic Psychology

FOCUS indicates the complexity of scientific researches that have gone nto the development of Quontic Psychology.

organism. In the center ring are three aspects of the person continually affected by all the feedback from the six sides of the cube. At the same time that the cube sides are fields of study they also represent parts of environment-self interactions that play roles in the formation of the personality of the human being. Feedback going back and forth between the cube sides to the organic self, consciousness and memory in the central ring continually alters personal experience. Although the sides of the cube in the diagram are separated in three-dimensional space, it must be understood that in a wholistic understanding of nature nothing is actually separate from anything else and all these cube sides continually interact in consciousness and in the behaving person. Through consciousness we are able to both receive and return to our awareness of and connection with all of nature.

Looking at the center of the cube a little while will enable the viewer to see the ring in the center as floating and the cube itself may shift perspectives. It is a way to represent the dynamic and continually shifting nature of the interactions among all the parts of a person's life.

The fields of study represented on the cube will be more or less kept separate in what follows, but their interwoven relationships will be continually pointed out.

This massive conceptual integration that is being proposed, that is, the sciences with each other, the individual with the effects introjected from his environment through their mutual interactions, the individual with the processes of nature and of course, the individual within himself can't be understood without a guiding principle big enough to facilitate its accomplishment. Such a guiding principle must be comprehensive enough to function in all of nature as well as in the sciences and still be critical for the maintainance of human life, It must also ultimately have some way to be connected with the paranormal dimension, since that is what we wish to integrate with all the others.

I wish to suggest that such a broadly encompassing need and purpose is fulfilled by the Homeostatic Principle. The understanding of this principle is what will be fleshed out in the next several chapters. This will be adequate to prepare the reader for the basic concepts behind the model of Quontic Psychology which I've developed for the specific integration of relationships between what will be called third dimensional and fifth dimensional energies. I will draw on empirical research in the sciences, phenomenological research in the psychology of normal, abnormal and paranormal human functioning and concepts in Eastern mysticism toward this end. Finally, given the complexity of the subject, I will attempt to keep it as simple, clear, and interesting as possible.

Consciousness

"Painting, for me, when it really 'happens' is as miraculous as any natural phenomenon—as, say, a lettuce leaf. By 'happens' I mean the painting in which the inner aspect of man and his outer aspects interlock....The painting I have in mind, painting in which inner and outer are inseparable, transcends technique, transcends subject and moves into the realm of the inevitable—then you have the lettuce leaf."

— Artist, Lee Krasner

The Miraculous Mystery of the Lettuce Leaf

The concept of FOCUS introduced in the last chapter will undoubedly provoke skepticism in many people. It is a new way of looking at phenomena, violating the customary and comfortable attitudes into which people sink. It means trying to understand and integrate matters which appear too mysterious and too diverse to ever be understood, no less related. And that is precisely why it is also so intriguing to pursue it. Mystery creates its own energy which synergizes the lettuce leaf.

Within each person also lies a mystery, enormous, promising and profound. The questions provoked by the mystery of the inner self may never adequately be resolved. With the information explosion from scientific, paranormal, and computerized techniques, new questions follow new information, spreading like the ripples of a pebble in a pond. Some people throw their pebbles into it, and to find answers they search out different directions; some take up psychotherapy, some take up esoteric studies and philosophy, some become professional or amateur scientists; others may feel it's sufficient to simply live and let the mysteries take care of themselves. Many feel the questions provoked by new and puzzling information, but deny and reject it out of fear. Fear is what makes change so difficult, fear of the unknown in oneself as well as out there.

Even though it may appear untouchable without risking dire consequences, fear can be understood and dissipated. Becoming afraid will happen to people who are open to exploring the unknown. The mystery of the unknown, drawing people like a magnet, at the same time repulses people because of the feeling of danger. It is a grown up version of a child sleeping in a dark room. For a child, the parameters of the self are not known and the potentials in the real world are often felt as threatening to survival. In today's world, danger is unfortunately more realistic and fear among children is more widespread than ever. The secure boundaries of home and family and the safety of one's school and neighborhood are often invaded, if not gone.

By the time one reaches adulthood a person has negotiated his life through all these dangerous shoals of potential catastrophe and believes he knows himself and enough about reality to navigate safely through its storms. If he is then drawn toward the unknown, irrational, unexplained aspect of the universe and of himself, he then faces the potentials of opening up feelings of anxiety that were once dealt with or suppressed. For the inquiring, exploring adult, continuing the search for the nature of reality becomes tied to fear of changing one's perceptions of a self that is intimately related to conditioned developmental relationships with preconceptions about reality.

The self-concept, like the ego and like reality, is a product of a developmental process. How we perceive ourselves is due to the interactions that take place during our years of growth and development. Often, during infancy and child-hood we had feelings that we expressed for which we received rewards or punishments, so we learned that we were right or wrong and good or bad, strong or weak, depending on different behaviors — "brave boys don't cry" and "good girls just listen". Those rewards and punishments were feedback systems that turned into our self-concepts of when and how we are good and bad, which - sometimes contrary to our intentions - remains with us the rest of our lives. To comply with the rewards and punishments we separated good and bad behaviors out from each other, and repressed those that would not be rewarded. This kind of attempt at homeostasis with the self in relation to the developmental environment demanded a sacrifice which sabotaged the alternative goal - also demanded by parents and teachers - of truthfulness. And punishment for any reason only created more fear and served to further destroy the connections with the organic, fundamentally homeostatic growth of self.

As children it seemed that we had little choice but to accept fragmenting ourselves into parts that were good, bad, loving, angry etc., and repressing the punishable thoughts and feelings as a way of learning to cope.   By and for this fragmentation we were, and certainly are still, manipulated and conditioned, by ourselves as well as others, into continu-ing a self-concept that receives further good rewards for sabotaging its own organically based awareness. However, making choices is crucial to our health and well-being.

As children, giving up choices becomes a pragmatically useful way of relating to the conditioning of society. Giving up choices produces gains in security, good grades that can lead to good jobs, success in a conforming social system that is, in principle though not in practice, oiled to perform efficiently as possible. Sometimes, if the noose is too tight, the price for conventional security is a self-constriction paid for with various types of psychophysiological illness and/or emotional problems.

The other side of this argument is that we are not islands unto ourselves and need each other to satisfy needs. Therefore, relationships demand adjustments of one sort or another. We discover there is a homeostasis, a sense of balance and well-being that comes from satisfying interpersonal relationships. However, many have found that this homeostatic sense is not dependent on compliant relationships—it functions best on contact with inner knowledge. An inner sense of homeostasis inevitably guides the person more sensitively than anything or anyone else can. It is continually amazing to me how wisely the self functions to offer the connections needed to the unconscious to heal the complicated anguish of adults, even that which began in childhood.

Sybil at the Beginning of Therapy

The example of Sybil is presented in two parts. The first is a general review of her problems as they developed in the first months of therapy. The second is an example of a session which was a fine example of how she made a connection with her inner homeostasis which helped her with the anguish in her childhood.

Sybil complained, sometimes with a whine, that she was angry but didn't know why. It was terrible because she was angry at her boy friends—usually more than one simultaneously, angry at coworkers and angry at herself. She didn't want to hurt anyone so she controlled herself—the mechanism was that of blaming herself for being angry and not knowing why. She functioned well intellectually, was logical and rational, polite and kind to people so she could maintain a modicum of interpersonal relationship. But she was continually fatigued, could not find a direction or a way to work that satisfied her, and whatever she did she felt unsuccessful. She had paranormal experiences she could not explain and was interested in finding out more about them. Her love life was also unsatisfying, especially with men her own age. Why was she that way, always angry and unhappy, unable to establish a firm relationship with a man, especially one that could offer her security in marriage?.

A little exploration revealed she continually berated herself for not being successful while another part of her wanted to lay back, relax, take it easy and explore herself spiritually. A look at her parents showed that her father was very successful but emotionally unavailable while her mother criticized her, made her feel like a failure and drove her continually to accomplish more. Her mother was a housewife, frustrated at having to give up the stage to marry her father. Her parents were continually in conflict or they avoided each other. Even when he was home her father was not available for contact, though she seemed to have a vague memory of being special to him during infancy. As she grew older, Sybil identified with her mother uncritically and rejected her father as her mother did. In that way she didn't have to find the hurt, anger and rejected needs she felt at his unavailability.

There was no attempt by either parent to find out who she was, what she felt, or to have her develop goals that came out of her own organic being. Because her survival was tied to her mother, she overlooked and repressed any and all her negative feelings toward her. She didn't dare feel the rejection, hurt and anger coming from the conditional love so rarely bestowed for being successful, or hurt by the mockery of her spiritual ideas. Now she finds that her relationship to her own organic needs and spiritual truths are demeaned by this introjected mother because the organic and spiritual parts of her conflict with becoming successful and prevent her from fulfilling her mother's idealized model.

However, on the other hand, if she succeeds in ways that her mother has failed, she will run the risk of being successful like her father and rejected by her mother. She was trapped, tied up in knots, caught, imprisoned in a catch-22. Her mother, she thought, was already jealous of the slight successes she had already attained.

Comments and Ruminations

No wonder she felt herself "tied up in knots". Little wonder, too, without the fundamental experience of a loving father and with lifelong training to hate men, she could not establish a strong heterosexual relationship.

The organic truth is expressed in her bodily feelings: a gut tied up in knots and fatigued. She is repeatedly sick and is afraid of coming down with cancer. The anger that is tied up and creating the fatigue is detached from her mother and father and given an unkown but frightening externalized source, mostly to protect the maternal relationship. The direction that would come from her organically real and spiritual self is not accepted because it means a shift in what reality is about in her self, and a moving away from parental training and her family values.

Underneath the socially induced reality of the developmental years lies buried the potential for an appreciation of the self and of the world beyond social conditioning. Knowing reality as it might have been had it not been fragmented and thus destroyed is too dangerous for adults as well as for children. It is not surprising that some people need psychotherapeutic help in order to understand and unblock themselves in their search for physical and mental health, while simultaneously searching for a larger truth.

Returning to a description of the pitfalls and dragons we faced during our childhood enables us to understand what kind of adults we are. Our adulthood is psychophysiologically simply a continuation of our childhood, with a few added complications and disguises.

Starting in childhood and continuing in adulthood, we put on several layers of skin that become a way of thinking and feeling about ourselves that we project toward the outer world. Thus in the earliest years is born our defense system, learning at a very early age to adopt those facades that will be most effective in achieving parentally directed goals.

What the skin protects becomes buried in our unconscious memory in a real self that is blocked from becoming ex-

pressed. Sybil's pain and anger are not honestly directed
against her misguided parents but become abstracted, objec-
tified into fear of cancer. Emotions are not wiped out, they
are simply stored out of sight to prevent them from acting
in a way that may threaten her conditioned control over her
behavior. Defense mechanisms, from childhood on, work to
develop what is considered at the time to be a livable reality
while distorting it. Unfortunately, we don't realize just how
much these layers of defenses shape our view of the feelings
we perceive in others and our view of the world. When our
layers of skin are very thick we may have to distort reality
considerably to collaborate with and confirm the values
promoted by our frightened, defended selves.

There is a certain amount of tolerance within the
psychodynamic system for compromises which will nevertheless maintain the healthy functioning of the system as a
whole. At the same time that a livable balance is sought with
the external environment, there is in everyone a psychophysiological knowledge of homeostasis that functions, to
some degree, independently of the responses of the world
around us. The sense of internal balance is thrown off by
dystonic interpersonal energies when disruptions are very
powerful - such as during traumatic parental and love relationships. Then the strain and stress of maintaining itself
shows up as illness on physical as well as psychological levels.

The job of therapy is to help stabilize the ship so that it
can rock without capsizing. To do this takes the opening up
of contact with the inner self of homeostatic energies.

A Session with Sybil One Year Later

She said she felt - uh, strange - having to come into a
session and say something. She always had to begin. It was
a strange relationship she had with me. She didn't know
what to say. It wasn't social, it wasn't a friendship, it was all
about her. Wasn't I bored listening to people's problems?
How could I stand it session after session? She was afraid

she would probably say the wrong thing, mess it up, she'd fall on her face. She knew she had a lot of fear tying her up. She felt as if she were paralyzed.

I told her she sounded as if she were right at home. She agreed, it was the kind of criticism she had to listen to from her mother. It would be similar from her father as well when he talked to her.

She looked soft and vulnerable, different a bit. In response to my questions, she said she had a lot of energy, didn't know what to do with it. It was in her stomach. No, she didn't want to talk to it but she would lay down and do a relaxation exercise. I gave her a deep breathing relaxation, to expel toxic energy and take in fresh, nutritious air and "feel it in all the organs of your body." Then I asked for her imagery.

First she was in a dark place, then she developed an image of being on a mountaintop, a clear view all around her, relaxing and refreshing.

I asked her to imagine and connect with an idealized mother. She saw this earthy woman, heard her telling her that she cared about her and loved her. Now she felt like a child, wanted to sit on her lap and embrace her, which she did. She said to the mother she was grateful for her support and loved her as well. How was her stomach, I asked?

Yes, she also still felt the tension around and in her stomach. She let it speak out. It wanted to jump up and down, yell and scream. When she focussed in on it, it was a need for a man. Then it was a need for her father and then a sexual feeling toward him. Was it normal? I assured her it was. Then why did it take her so long to feel it - she demanded of herself? Most people never ever let themselves feel it, I said, its too threatening, too contrary to the taboo. She was doing great and needed to give herself time. She relaxed into it again, acknowledged it was like her feeling toward a boy friend, much older than herself. She wanted to embrace her father. She took a pillow, folded her arms around it and spoke loving words, then bade him farewell.

When she sat up she felt calm, she said, her stomach was fine, she was connected with her body and centered. There was a lovely look on her face, and as she thanked me we wished each other a good week and she left.

Further Comments

The first sessions, early in her therapy, were based on Sybil's childhood upbringing and the distortions, blockages, and frustrations that were imposed and integrated from her family's values. That set the stage for the false homeostasis which is unstable, a superficially stable state that doesn't satisfy the real homeostatic needs of the child or the grownup that she will become.

A dehomeosis can't remain that way without caving in sooner or later to its own pressures, either in physical or mental illness. Her fear of cancer, which was not borne out, may have nevertheless been a prognostic awareness that this - or some other deadly illness - is what would occur if she didn't take corrective action. The anxiety in that sense was helpful in giving her the information that she was in danger of something worse. That "something worse" did not have to materialize as long as she was informing herself regarding the causes of the dehomeosis so that she could bring herself into a unifunctional way of perceiving and relating to herself and others.

What the second session demonstrates is how a homeostatic state is the outcome of interactions that can occur between psychological, physiological and paranormal inputs. After she received the love from the fantasied earth mother, a source of nourishment accessible from within herself, she felt her need for a male love object and could express that need somewhat as a child would have, which she would never have dared do in her actual childhood. The separation of sexuality as a felt experience from loving interactions between parents and children further fragments and represses the potential for wholeness. As a result, these repressed feelings may return in a physically dysphoric form as perverted sexuality including pedophilia and child abuse. At the opposite end, adults report false "memories" of sexual abuse. They fantasize their parents or parent surrogates have acted out their own repressed childhood sexual fantasies. Giving Sybil permission to have this feeling toward her father then enabled her to give it up and ultimately to move into a better relationship with a man her own age.

Maya in Science

This, to me, is the meaning of "Maya" in Eastern mystical philosophy: That we live with socially induced illusions about reality, negative as well as positive, that have been conditioned into us or are the outcome of unconscious events during our development while true reality remains unknown.

There are very few truths that have held up through the ages. Each society creates its own truths, as does each family and each individual. Science's claim on reality is just as subject to "Maya" as that of any individual. The totality of it may be ultimately unknowable in any but an intuitive sense, but, at the same time that it feels like a risk, the search is always alluring and energizing to the person's sense of who he is and who he might be and might still become.

Contemporary psychology has demonstrated through many psychological, social and perceptual studies that distortions of reality are commonplace, that "objective reality" is disguised by defense mechanisms or distorted by perceptual and emotional processes. Thinking, which is considered a fundamentally logical, objectively oriented process, often actually follows psychodynamic, perceptual and emotional, or defensive priorties. These priorities are rooted in body and mind, our personal unseen universe.

Thought itself is frequently determined by the psychodynamics of neurosis, that is, of the distortions of a system dangerously skewed away from its own normal, organic, homeostatic range. We will find that homeostasis is a principle that runs equally through mundane, scientific and spiritual parts of the self-environment dynamic. The striving for it creates a motivation for the homeostatic energy. It is coupled with survival and determines a great deal of organic, interpersonal, scientific and spiritual behavior. It is also the golden thread that ties together the functions of the various components of the quontic psychological system.

However, the guiding principle of homeostasis itself can be thrown into disarray by the effects of Maya - longstanding systemic psychophysiological distortions. Sickness is the signal, like the red light on the dash of a car, that the system is badly off balance or is missing something it needs to continue running well. When this happens, the contents of consciousness have to be open to question and change if a person is to resume healthy physical and emotional functioning.

Consciousness is an integral part of homeostatic functions. They work hand in glove to promote survival of the human being and of the human race. We can't be sure this partnership will succeed because it depends on how well it is steered, how badly the ship was off course or how far along on its way toward capsizing. Can it be brought back into balance?

We think that being realistic is the way to steer the ship toward homeostasis. However, reality is finally a subjective experience, as we are beginning to see, even in the "hard" science of physics. If everyone agreed on what reality was all about there would be no conflicts or wars or divergent theories about how the cosmos works; good and bad, right and wrong would be the same for everyone. Difficult as that is, rigidity would be even worse. Reality, when it becomes a rigid, hard, inflexible system is contrary to and opposed to the drive we have to gain a homeostatic means of survival.

This inflexibility, in the hands of authority and expertise, is the danger that the "hard" sciences of physics and medicine are currently facing. Being able to change one's view of reality can only happen if a person, especially a scientist, is bravely committed to a consciousness that questions itself deeply, thereby changing and broadening its perception of self and of the world around.

Therefore, I do not use scientific discoveries in traditionally scientific ways. Once I find something I do not stop at the scientific statement but often go far beyond it to see what might be the implications that the traditional scientist would deny. Or, as has also happened frequently much to my surprise, I will speculate on some dynamic intuitively first and come up with some concept only to discover an experiment or a concept in a scientific journal or book that appears to support what I have intuited.

We are all discovering the same truths about reality simultaneously. This to me is the interlocked workings of the inner and outer energies so beautifully expressed in the lettuce leaf metaphor for a painting, offered by Lee Krasner above. It's the Homeostatic Principle at work. This principle is more than human and practical. It runs through everything, it is universal, therefore it is also spiritual, connecting all of our immense resources for knowledge. Describing how they interrelate, to return to unity from fragmentation is what Quontic Psychology is about.

As it grew, I wanted to develop a model which could serve as a roadmap for the voyage to the fifth dimension. To do this, I had to first take into account the mundane three dimensional characteristics of psychophysiological functions in everyday life. Too many spiritual models try to bypass contemporary, mundane reality by ignoring the tremendous importance and impact of developmental and current experience. We have to understand ourselves better on this level before turning to higher level fifth dimensional modes of functioning. After that, I could look at the way in which science as well as intuition offered insightful concepts that could assist in building a unitary system.

The next chapter presents a psychoneurological model showing the way psyche and soma interact to form consciousness. This is followed with an Eastern metaphysical model of consciousness, and the two of them are compared.

Models of Consciousness

"The world is full of paradox. For example, [in Buddhism] though no notion of a creator is entertained, great stress is laid upon the need for faith and piety. By faith is meant not trust in a benevolent deity avid for love, praise and obedience, but conviction that, beyond the seeming reality misreported by our senses which is inherently unsatisfactory, lies a mystery which, when intuitively perceived, will give our lives undreamed-of meaning and endow the most insignificant object with holiness and beauty."

— John Blofeld, <u>Gateway to Wisdom</u> [1]

Psychoneurological Consciousness

Consciousness research has come a long way, but it is by no means finished. Neurological research has developed theories explaining how consciousness is the outcome of physiological structures (John 1976 [2]). Some physicists have begun to solve systemic and practical dilemmas by calling on consciousness to explain gaps in scientific theory. Some paleontologists have been looking at the idea of an evolution in consciousness.

Or is it the other way around, and as the Eastern philosophies say, the source of all life is in consciousness, therefore it is represented in all the multiplicity of forms that make up our environment as well as ourselves? There is no ready answer to that dilemma. We will first examine what a neurophysiologist has to say.

The neurophysiological point of view of Dr. E. Roy John, Director of the Brain Research Labs at N.Y.U. Medical Center, represents a physiological position that fits into the quontic psychological paradigm most readily. It constitutes a neuropsychological grounding for a survival-oriented motivation in behavior. The survival aspect will become clear when we take up the research of Dr. Jonathon Winson in the next chapter. However, consciousness also has a meta-physical component which has to become integrated with its psychophysiological base in human behavior.

With a fundamentally empirical point of view, Dr. John believes that in order to include all that which constitutes consciousness, it is necessary to begin at the most basic levels of neurological and biochemical organismic structures. However, the totality of consciousness, and of personality, goes beyond the contributions of specific neurological structures to form a Gestalt that cannot be found in the constituents of the body's individual and separate parts. Therefore, what forms the link between physiological structures and the larger whole that becomes consciousness, subjective experience, self, self-awareness and finally mind? Neurological paths form patterns that interlink the individual parts through neuronal, electromagnetic and biochemical connections, and it is through the interactions of the linked relationships of these patterns that consciousness emerges. In the neurological point of view, consciousness is an emergent structure reflecting a physiological process, not a causal one as it is in Eastern mysticism.

John proposes that mind arises from six levels or orders of information. They are repeated at length here, and expanded upon, because they form the physiological counterpart of the psychological functioning of consciousness which was described in some detail in the last chapter. Although dating back to 1976, this work coming out of neurophysiological research is also the most clear counterpart of what occurs in psychotherapy, and in a sense in all holistic therapies, today. John's six levels are as follows:

1. SENSATIONS:

Consciousness is an information network of psychoneurological sensations or impulses stimulated by the "irritability of living matter" to make adjustments to the environment, at its simplest level.

We will see later that this "irritability of living matter" may well be the stress aspect of a survival process, which, in the resulting need to solve survival problems, drove the evolution of both brain and consciousness toward the form in which we see and know them today. We will also examine how genetic inheritance of solutions to survival problems possibly led to an overall guidance schemata in DNA.

Consciousness, after all is said and done, is recognized in Quontic Psychology as the greatest and perhaps most complex human homeostatic, feedback, survival mechanism yet evolved in the great pantheon of nature's trials and errors. In its earliest stages it begins in primitive life with inputs from a network of physical sensations coming from biochemical and electromagnetic processes that go through an association and organizational hierarchy evolving into ever greater complexity to become consciousness.

2. PERCEPTIONS:

Perception is the faculty of making "...interpretations of the meaning of sensations in the context of stored information about previous experiences...information resulting from an interaction between sensations and memories." (John 1976, P.3) (Our underline)   Later, he says, "...Cerebral events, termed readout or emitted potentials,...reflect the generation of processes corresponding to the memory of past or imaginary stimuli." (John 1976, P. 16)

The past merges through its memories with the present in perception. In addition, we might add that all living matter has memory in a broad sense. The genetic code of organic life in its DNA carries in itself the brand of that organism's inheritance which enables it to reproduce itself. On the evolutionary scale then, physiological memory at the level of the smallest cells, the amoebas and planktons, is present. Physiological memories combine with sensations to give rise to perceptions which in turn may produce new "irritations" - stressfully felt conditions - which give rise to new problem-solving adaptations which in turn result in new psychophysiological memories encapsulated in DNA. New research being conducted currently supports the probability that memories are an aspect of the genetic code which surface psychologically as well as physiologically in the human organism. How far back in time can evolutionary memories go?

My underlined statement impinges on the psychodynamics of integrating ideas of consciousness with physiology, and implicates past life therapy as well. This is further expanded in the next, third order or level of information.

3. CONSCIOUSNESS:

"...a process in which information about multiple individual modalities of sensation and perception is combined into a unified, multidimensional representation of the state of the system and its environment and is integrated with information about memories and the needs of the organism, generating emotional reactions and programs of behavior to adjust the organism to its environment....The content of consciousness is the momentary constellation of these different types of information....Memories are activated, attention is focused, perceptions influenced, emotions aroused, drive priorities altered, and plans of behavior revised as a result of...feedback, producing a continuous reorganization of basic processes because of the influence of higher level integrative and analytical functions." (John 1976, P.4)

A more complete statement than the above about the operation of memories and consciousness in the quontic system as used in Organic Process Therapy could hardly be formulated. Psychotherapy, to be effective, has to reflect living organisms by being a multidimensional process. It reaches into neurological communications systems that interact with the self-image and the ego to formulate perceptions. These perceptions, sensations and emotions participate with activated memories, unconsciously as well as preconsciously, to feed input to consciousness.

The interactive psychophysiological process begins when external stimuli generate neurological excitations—beginning in infancy, if not in the womb. (See Chapter 9 on "Dimensions of Time and Memory"). Psychoneurological responses become inputted and embedded through bioelectrochemical processes carried out by the neurological system. These patterned pathways become memories on a psychophysical bodymind level. As new events occur, these become matched up and integrated with feedback from embedded memories. Together with input from presently experienced needs, the resultant is fed into consciousness to become checked out with the ego, thus filling out the perceived reality of the immediate situation. Psychodynamically, the total resultant becomes the content of active consciousness.

It must be remembered that this is a neurophysiological paradigm we are presenting even though it is clearly suitable as a paradigm for psychotherapy. Nevertheless it lacks the inclusion of a paranormal or spiritual aspect. In Eastern philosophy, the paradigm would begin with Consciousness as The Great Causal Essence which animates matter out of which human material consciousness would arise.

If the question of memory and consciousness are seen from the point of view of science, then one must ask where and how early in the history of mankind did consciousness begin. Did a process of development from a simple physiological memory in a one-celled animal like a protozoa change into sensation-perceptual-psychological memory, to integrate into human consciousness in the course of evolution? There are researchers who believe that animals, particularly primates and dolphins (St. John 1991[3]), are capable of thought-like responses and therefore may be said to own consciousness. But, at present, there is no adequate definition of it. Nevertheless, the above questions will not be ignored.

To continue abstracting the neuropsychology of E.Roy John:

4. SUBJECTIVE EXPERIENCE:

Information from the contents of consciousness provides the fuel for subjective experience, but it is the tip of the iceberg. The quality of subjective experience is credited to the organization of lower level patterns which are very different from the quality of the discharge itself. Meaning is not inherent in the pattern, but is the experienced personal outcome of relevant organizational factors. Subjective experience serves to organize diverse multidimensional experiences into a continuous unity which gives the pattern personal meaning. Thus, in the experience itself, a person is not aware of all the multitude of neurological factors contributing to the experience, all he becomes aware of is the continuity available (through the match of unconscious past and consciously present information). For functional purposes, he is only aware of the meaning and significance of an experience to himself in the present moment, which constitutes a subjective experience. (1976, P. 5)

5. THE SELF:

The self is like a collation of one's personal history, the accumulated memories of sets of fourth order (subjective) information. The person's individual historical record of subjective memories and experiences coalesce into a framework and a concept called the Self.

We might ask here, briefly, whether the accumulated memories that coalesce into the self-concept could not have deep sources of input from an unconscious of past lives. Human evolution with its accumulation of genetic memories could include the memories of past lives.

6. SELF-AWARENESS:

"If we consider subjective experiences as higher-order sensations, then, self-awareness is analogous to the perception of those sensations." says John. Self-awareness is a kind of overview of the self in its integration of subjective experiences. Through self-awareness a person interprets present experience in conjunction and comparison with the pattern of previous subjective experiences from the conscious viewpoint of the self. It is as if a feedback loop is established between present and past stimuli which powerfully and continuously affect each other.

What is so interesting in John's work, and why I have quoted him so extensively, is that his source of information is neurological research, yet it parallels, supports, and at some points it clarifies observations that have been made by means of psychotherapy. It acknowledges that memories of early emotional events in this lifetime can be systematically recaptured psychodynamically in a psycho-neuro-physiological system. A biochemical, electromagnetic and neurological feedback system between aware consciousness and lower levels of body functioning facilitates this process. It is accompanied or followed by systematic, intentional, rational as well as unconscious searches for memories which give more continuity and meaning to life experiences. The psychotherapy process enables the result of these searches to be used beneficially to understand oneself better in relation to current experience.

Now, let's begin to examine consciousness as presented through a different Eastern point of view to find personality structures beyond the physical level that will help to integrate the physical and the transpersonal domains.

An Overview

E.R. John is anything but a mystic since he fundamentally says that consciousness is the outcome of association patterns developed biochemically and neurologically, and that there is a higher "subjective experience" that allows the self to be aware of consciousness, which is generated from the association patterns among themselves. This patterning generating a subjective experience permits a higher level of consciousness to emerge than the individual biochemical patterns would permit, but even with a lift onto a higher plane from the Gestalt concept, it is still no higher than the possibilities a basically materialistic scheme allows.

In the view of mystics, consciousness generates material reality, whereas in John's view (representative of the position of many open-minded, organically-oriented scientists) the neurological and biochemical activities of the body wholly generate consciousness. An opening to a higher but still non-mystical level is given in the Gestalt which is not definable by its parts alone. In the organic viewpoint, of which John's is an example, neurological-biochemical connections relate as patterns which create emotional and psychological connections among events which have occurred in the lifetime of the individual. Those connections occurring in a person's lifetime are distributed and accrued as familiar sensory stimuli into a system of memory distributions. And, we can add again, memory plays a focal part in consciousness.

I have taken another step and have suggested adding metaphysical aspects such as past lives into the system of psychophysiological and genetic memory distributions which are accrued and subject to rearousal under appropriate daily as well as therapeutic conditions. In doing so, the spiritual dimension is of necessity included, but not yet accounted for in a specific physiological context.

Any model of consciousness that attempts to explain and integrate human behavior must recognize that the functions of consciousness consolidates, evaluates, makes decisions, remembers, integrates, and attempts to make sense of, give meaning to, reality. Those functions of consciousness are, against our rational preferences, influenced by needs, values and belief systems and sometimes stimulated by fantasy and illusions.

All of that complex behavior is also guided by another part of mental functioning we call the ego. In general its function is to bring into responsive balance the needs, values, and feelings of the intrapersonal self with that of the extrapersonal stimulation we encounter in daily life. The way it accomplishes that in relation to the external environment is through the mediation of the perceptual and cognitive faculties. This, in turn, varies from person to person due to the uniqueness of each person's experiences and memories, so that there are many different kinds of ego systems and therefore many different kinds of responses to deal with in our interpersonal encounters.

A Buddhist Model

One of the ways in which I have come to expand my understanding of what role consciousness and the ego serve is by studying Buddhism, which I've now been doing for the past twenty years. What I find is that the Buddhists, beginning almost 2000 years ago, were describing ego functions that we are just becoming aware of and knowledgeable about today in the West. So let me present a brief summary of one Buddhist (different schools have different models just as in the West) model of consciousness.

This particular Buddhist model postulates nine levels of consciousness. The first five levels are the same as the five senses:
1. Vision
2. Hearing
3. Taste
4. Touch
5. Olfaction

The next four levels are specifically Buddhist:
6. Integration of Sensory Input.
7. Ego Awareness
8. Alaya Consciousness
9. Buddha-nature.

The last four levels are unfamiliar to Western Psychology (even #7 is unfamiliar due to the way it is used here) so they need to be amplified and explained.

6. INTEGRATION OF SENSORY INPUT:

This level can be compared to what we call the synthesizing function of the thinking process. It serves to screen and organize data for meaningfulness so that the myriad of disconnected impulses entering the sensorium can be either ignored or related to other, more familiar data. In Western neuro-psychology we have seen a similar psychophysiological organization of sensory input in John's system. In that system the outcome is consciousness and self-awareness. In this respect, Eastern and Western models overlap.

7. EGO AWARENESS:

It ought to be easy for us to accept and understand this level, but there is a vast gap in the manner in which Eastern and Western Psychology relate to the ego. For the mystics, the ego is basically non-substantial, an artifact of human development that needs only to be recognized for its own small part and not be attributed over-importance as it is in Western psychology where it has acquired the same significance as the whole person.

When Buddhists talk about ego they are talking about an aspect of mind which is an illusion we created to manage our daily affairs whose centrality disappears when the true nature of reality is understood. "It is a function of self which is like a monkey on a string made to dance to the tune, so to speak, of the Alaya consciousness". (Nozaki 1984 [4])

8. ALAYA CONSCIOUSNESS:

This is the storehouse or accumulation of all the person's Karma (the result of all those unresolved past lives) as well as those actions performed from the time of birth in this lifetime up to the present moment. This obviously may cover many centuries, a concept which is as alien to Western psychology as it is familiar and comfortable to Eastern psychology. The expanded, broadest implication is that we all carry within us evolutionary knowledge of every aspect of human, if not cosmic, growth and development at a deep, unconscious level of mind. It is comparable to what is called "the Akasic Record" or the Quontic Warehouse described in the next section.

The Ego and the Alaya

The Alaya consciousness carries a double weighted value, it is a two-edged sword. Not only can it carry its knowledge about existence from Karma into the ego awareness level of consciousness, but it may also be severely distorted by the ego's input to the reality function. This means that, filtered through the Ego, Karma itself may include defense and distortion mechanisms which affect a person's current life experience.

In both Eastern and Western psychologies, the ego awareness level is a function that is committed to dealing realistically and effectively with the here-and-now of experience. In so doing, it must be continually receiving, evaluating, accepting or rejecting stimuli from both the internal and the external environment. It may set up goals of action and standards of behavior for itself which we call character. To be realistic, a person must also be able to learn from experience and change the way he behaves when appropriate or necessary.

However, the ego also responds to and reflects the level of Integration of Sensory Input (6) in its responses to stimuli. Level 6 is neurologically as well as developmentally dependent on internally developed interoceptive processes. There is a continual interplay between internal and external stimuli occurring in the human organism, an interplay which is not modest in its capacity for change in perceptual and cognitive responses. This can include past lives in Karmic Theory.

9. BUDDHA-NATURE:

Last is cosmic-consciousness or Buddha-nature. We can't reasonably expect to reach the ninth layer in one lifetime, but at least it's there for anyone adventurous enough to establish that goal for the sake of taking the hero's journey. It's reward is a consciousness of cosmic life force in which the realm of the self is coextensive with the universe and possesses all the phenomena and all the energies of the universe within itself consciously. Of course, reaching this layer can only be achieved by ridding oneself of the delusions and the distortions of consciousness at the level of ego awareness, thus cleansing it of the neuroticism which makes up the Maya of experience. In attaining the ninth level the person joins his energy into the cosmic forces of wisdom, freedom, compassion and enlightenment. The following Yogic prayer gives a succinct sense of the path to follow for enlightenment:

"I and all sentient beings from beginningless time have been involved in the creation of many kinds of evil karma-forming activity obstructive of Enlightenment. Ignorant of the Buddhas and of the Way to Liberation, we have wandered through repeated births and deaths without knowledge of the marvellous principles enunciated by Shakyamuni Buddha. Now in the presence of the Bodhisattva of Compassion and the Buddhas of the ten quarters of the universe, I (or we) express remorse on behalf of all living beings for these failings, desiring only to assist them in overcoming hindrances to Enlightenment." (Blofield 1980)

Comparison of John, Western and Alaya Consciousness

Alaya consciousness can, from the perspective of interactions of internal and external stimuli, be seen to be conceived along similar lines as the neurophysiological structure of consciousness developed out of his research by E. Roy John. However, there is the fundamental difference that the Alaya may go back many lifetimes whereas the consciousness of E.R. John stays within this lifetime.

In dynamic, regressive psychotherapies such as Organic Process Therapy, it is recognized that the interplay of life experience has a powerful effect on the ego's way of seeing the here-and-now, the present moment. For dynamic therapies, neurological and psychological structures are built on the foundations of early learning, (some believe as early as pre-birth), and the Eastern psychologies believe that learning is even screened and influenced by past lives.

The dynamic Western psychophysiologies have a common ground in the scientific research of neurology, and as we shall see later, the transpersonal, fifth dimensional domain receives a contribution from controversial concepts in physics. We will also turn to an examination of the neurobiological concepts of Candace Pert and others to trace the specific part biochemistry may play in contemporary and genetic contributions to the evolution of consciousness and behavior.

For most conventional Western therapy, the ego has the most important place in personality functions, therefore Freud's famous dictum "Where Id was there shall Ego be" (Freud 1943 [5]). For Eastern and dynamic psychology it's level 8 or Alaya consciousness which plays the tune to which the other two levels, Ego Awareness and Integration of Sensory Input (also Jung 1964 [6]), must dance. My position is that the ego is an important reality testing device, but it cannot be maintained at the expense of the organic or real self without damage to the entire organism if it doesn't have an organic homeostatic basis. The end result could be a destructive lack of connection with the real, homeostatic issues of one's life and behavior. Whether or not the ego becomes destructive may also depend on the degree to which the content of the Alaya consciousness (including past lives) is permitted access to the reality testing ego function.

Thus, as in most psychotherapeutic schemata, when the ego is fed unwanted information from the Sensory and the Alaya levels which threatens the person's ego-oriented self-image in the here-and-now, then repression and its allied defense mechanisms will control the situation so as to maintain the status quo. For instance, as is so common among men who relate competitively, instead of acknowledging pain and hurt they will more easily distort it and show indifference or angry feelings as a generic sort of response. Being aggressive and competitively hostile is a socially accepted response among men whereas showing pain, fear, and crying are considered effeminate. So the feelings will be presented in a distorted way in order to preserve the self-image of masculine strength and mastery. On the other hand, the traditionally accepted view of "ladylike" behavior is to never display anger or aggression so these are distorted into crying, weakness, and victimization. Of course, the women's movement is changing all that. However, even within the two different genders, the specific triggers and mechanisms that provoke the ego to preserve the self-image under stressful conditions may differ because they are dependent on the personal history of the individual.

The most awesome representation of the capacity of the ego to distort reality in order to serve a compensated value system was put on view by Adolf Hitler and his need for superiority. Through his one way vision screen his ego could perform the most abominable acts imaginable, convince a whole nation it was also right to do it, and be proud of his accomplishments. This is what happens in smaller ways to everyone in the course of "normal" development. The ego sets up a one way vision screen to protect itself from further injury and pain and develops compensatory mechanisms for old fears and inadequacies after it has suffered painful assaults during the early years of development.

The same distortion or blocking is just as likely to be true of responses to stimuli coming from a past life source if it threatens to enter the here-and-now, so conscious knowledge of the Alaya will again be repressed. This can happen even while the Sensory and Alaya levels are affecting behavior because people become ingenious in manipulating their emotions to make them look like something else to themselves and to others.

In Western society, unlike the Eastern and some South American societies, the idea that we may have past lives is an "unrealistic" point of view. There's been an attempt to deal with this by past life therapist-researchers such as Dr. Helen Wambach (1984 [7]), Ian Stevenson (1974 [8]) and other very competent psychologists. As a society, we are not brought up in this kind of religious or metaphysical thinking and do not advocate this notion to others in bringing up their children. Nevertheless it is often noted that children have a naturally more metaphysical outlook than adults which gets drummed - or humdrummed out of them - when they become adults.

In effect, the metaphysical becomes repressed at an early age in our materialistic kind of reality. This means it becomes buried in the deeper layers of the unconscious along with the other threatening thoughts and feelings of children by the "realistic" guardianship mentality of the adult. Careful documentation of a case of a child who recounted the details of a former life as an adult which was checked out for accuracy and thus verified was published in 1980 in Brazil (Andrade 1980[9]). This particular case, called "The Case of Jacira and Ronaldo", was researched by a team at the Brazilian Institute for Psychobiophysical Research where fifty other cases have also been investigated and corroborated as to their facts in varying degrees.   Many hundreds of others have been researched by Ian Stevenson, an American investigator.

As a result of repression and its attendant defense mechanisms, "Maya" becomes "reality", a distortion of the truth. This distortion goes on through many cultures in many different ways. The outcome is that the Alaya consciousness remains intact and undisturbed with all its own distortions and repressions and consequent anguish. Thus, all the past lives we have lived as well as the emotional contortions we've created to survive in this one are passed into and repressed in the unconscious. This deeply disturbing unconscious material becomes feedback for the ego integration level. Current happenings with their new distortions are fed back into Alaya.

This is, in Eastern terms, how the Maya or illusions about reality are created in consciousness and is therefore what we have to overcome before we can gain access to a true picture of reality. More accurately, we must say we need to regain access to a reality with which we were once familiar.

No wonder they say it will take many lifetimes! And no wonder individual psychotherapy can be compared to an archeological excavation which can take a long time to unearth its wares until all its treasures are revealed.

Further Comparison of Eastern and Western Psychologies

In Western Psychology it is generally thought that the strength of the ego, its determination or vulnerability, passivity, rigidity or flexibility, is the biggest part of the problem for a person who wants to understand and make changes in behavior and deal better with reality. The way to deal with this life and its ongoing challenges and problems is, in the Western mode, to control one's emotions and develop a sophisticated and worldly ego.

More recently, Primal and rebirthing therapy have attempted to establish the content of infantile and birth trauma as the major concern of the therapy process.(Janov 1970) However, Primal which was popularized by Arthur Janov was limited in its reach since it did not, as is true of most other Western therapies, acknowledge the possibility of the existence of past lives or of a spiritual dimension. For Western psychology to accept past lives requires an expansion of the concept of the ego beyond Western limitations. The conventional American Psychological Association for instance is not able to go that far and has rejected Transpersonal Psychology as a Division member. However, there is a growing number of transpersonal and past life organizations and therapists here, such as the Association for Past Life Research and Therapies and the American Society for Psychical Research, which believe that the expansion is necessary. Otherwise we cannot do justice to the full range and potential of human experience.

In transpersonal psychology, the ego can seek an expansion of its awareness and knowledge by exploring the perimeters of the psychologically unknown and unfamiliar as well as by stretching its contact with the physically known universe. The growing Ego does not have to be opposed to Id (unintegrated drive energies), or Karma or Past Lives, it doesn't have to control the unknown in order to survive, as it does in conventional psychology. It needs to be open to the growth potentials inherent in accepting and integrating new awarenesses, new energies and new knowledge that is available to it - from the other-worldly, spiritual, as well as the worldly domains.

Worldly words filtered through the ego have become forms that create paradigms to feed illusions. This is done by an unreal ego. We must, once we have grown beyond childhood conditioning, transcend the unreal ego and its self-aggrandized illusions in order to fulfill our real nature within the non-illusion of true reality. In that sense, the adult is too often an illusion we create to protect and avoid the child within who is much closer to true reality. Recently, a winner in a drawing contest was announced and praised for his wonderful rendition of a tree. The winner turned out to be a four year old child whose mother sent in his drawing as a joke. We often laugh at the truth because its hard to take seriously, but recognize it unwittingly.

An adult person can maintain an ego that is secure and grounded in reality whose values and mode of functioning includes the spiritual dimension. Ego as a reality testing, searching, flexibly oriented system may place higher values on humanistic, growth, and environmentally conserving behaviors than on defensive, competitive, materialist kinds of priorities for behavior, and still remain a very adequate ego, achieving worldly success. It depends on what rewards you give yourself for what kinds of behavior and that is the outcome of a process which depends very much on social experience. Perhaps the ninth level of Buddha-nature will never be attained this way in Western culture, particularly since our society doesn't offer rewards or experientially known satisfactions for attaining Buddhahood, but a sufficiently intregrated ego which appreciates the necessity for both spiritual and daily human values can be harmoniously developed for great personal enhancement.

Unfortunately, most of the non-ego's basic sense of self and its ways of working are not known to consciousness. The non-ego, like consciousness and the mind as a whole, moves in ways that we cannot fixate, that we cannot place in a petri dish under a microscope; neither can we send it through a hole in a screen to count the number of marks it makes on our counting device. However, the work of the non-ego is manifest in everything, from the slightest movement (or lack of movement) to the most pronounced physical or verbal action that we take. It is inescapable, and it is what constitutes psychophysiological consciousness. It is ultimately the level that meets with mind to form a synergy that is fundamental to what we recognize as a human being.

Most contemporary science rejects the mind, and even consciousness, as a source of reliable information. I do not find that this is a tolerable situation. We will discuss consciousness as well as other aspects of mind repeatedly throughout the chapters of this book to find out what we may about the origins of consciousness, and to explore the way it operates within us. We will find that one of the ways in which consciousness is most crucial is to assist us in developing, maintaining and improving the character of homeostasis that governs our survival.

The Body-Mind at Work

"Evidence that theta rhythm encodes memories during REM sleep may be derived not only from neuroscientific studies but also from evolution."

— Jonathan Winson

The Immunolgical System in Memory, Storage and Transmission

If we are to understand the mind and consciousness, we have to understand how the bodymind operates in facilitating an internal communication system. We regard the body and mind as a "unifunctional" system, meaning they are one system in their mode of functioning in the human organism even though their origins may appear to be vastly different. The quontic model, which will be presented in the next chapter, incorporates all the interactions of the unifunctional bodymind with its incredible variety of input from genetic to transpersonal energies.

This system has many collaborators in somatopsychological processes of which only a minimal few can be described here. The human organism performs best through carrying out its grand-scale unifunctional and homeostatic functions. On the next page, Figure 7., *The Homeostatic Principle — Unifunctional Mind*, shows that the primary major thrust of consciousness in the quontic system is to insure survival using its inputs from experiential, psychological, paranormal and biological feedback to that end.

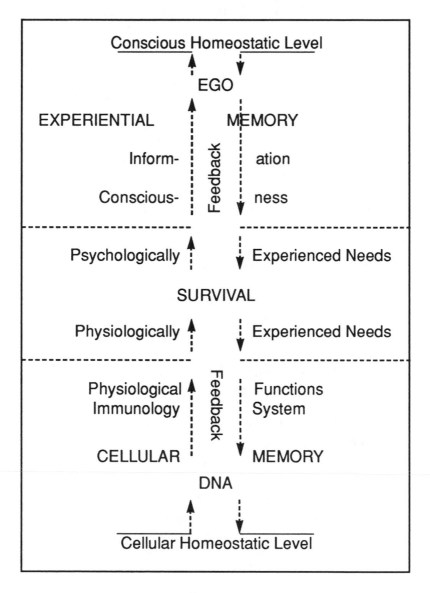

Figure 7.
The Homeostatic Principle — Unifunctional Mind,

shows that the primary major thrust of consciousness in the quontic system is to insure survival.

A fluid, well functioning communication system is basic to maintaining the homeostasis and survival of the body's organ systems. A poor mechanical analogy for human communication is the TV set which receives messages through its complicated mechanical circuitry and electrical sensitivity from a transmission center.

The human organism is a sensory receptive system but is not a TV set; among many other differences, we can transmit as well as receive messages. The communication problem in this analogy is that you know where the program originates within the transmission system in TV, but despite all the neurological research to date, we still can't say where feelings and memories are stored or where they originate in the body. Perhaps, we have to think, there is no physical or psychological place from which feelings and memories originate, not even within the brain. For some, that's a revolutionary idea.

We will see how memories are generated by a unifunctional process. There has been some recent research that clarifies and expands the physiological aspects of the storage, transmission and recall of memories, with their connection to emotions. In looking for what connects emotions to physiology, Candace B. Pert, formerly Chief of Brain Chemistry in the Clinical Neuroscience branch of the National Institutes of Mental Health, found that brain-body chemistry shows that neuropeptides are a key to that relationship. Her research shows that receptor cells abound in "nodal" or highly receptive areas of the body which communicate directly with peptide receptors in the brain. By creating a highly specialized network of neurochemical bonds, neurochemical carriers and receptors develop a system of information processing throughout the body, creating a "bodymind".

Pert states:

> "The striking pattern of neuropeptide receptor distribution in mood-regulating areas of brain, as well as their role in mediating communication throughout the whole organism, makes neuropep-

tides the obvious candidates for the biochemical mediation of emotion." (Pert 1986)[1]

This research reveals that ultimately neurochemicals are responsible for passing information between the rest of the body and the brain (which is obviously also part of the body). This network of neurochemical connectors pervades the limbic system, especially the hippocampus and the amygdala, which is the recognized brain-connected location serving the purpose of securing both emotional homeostasis and emotional communication in the person. (See the next diagram, Figure 8., *Brain and Spinal Cord*, major physiological components of body homeostasis.) There are additional nodal points outside the brain in the body which perform in the same manner as in the limbic system, and it therefore appears that emotions, via neurochemicals, actually pervade the entire human body as well as the brain.

The brain cannot operate without cooperation from the rest of the body of which it is a part. For instance, opiates such as morphine have their endogenous counterparts in body-produced pain relievers called beta-endomorphins. In addition to creating a state of calm, the endomorphins have also been recognized to have a healing effect on distressed body parts. Whether externally administered or produced internally, they operate in the same way, attaching to receptors throughout the body including the brain. Even the immunological system participates in this way in the bodymind activity of the neurochemical network. The integration of all these systems is so closely related, so intimate, it is no longer possible to separate body from brain, emotions from body and information from emotions, when viewed unifunctionally without the distortion of fragmentation. The entire bodybrain system is an intercommunication informational network. What informs the brain are bodymind sources of memory in addition to immediate stimuli. Information is what memory communicates and it's what makes consciousness so useful to homeostasis. Information is transmitted by the

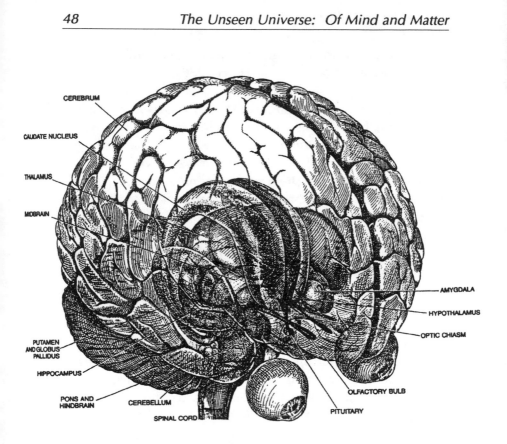

CEREBRUM

CAUDATE NUCLEUS

THALAMUS

MIDBRAIN

AMYGDALA

HYPOTHALAMUS

OPTIC CHIASM

PUTAMEN AND GLOBUS PALLIDUS

HIPPOCAMPUS

PONS AND HINDBRAIN

CEREBELLUM

OLFACTORY BULB

SPINAL CORD

PITUITARY

Figure 8.
Brain and Spinal Cord,

major physiological components of homeostasis.

The brain and spinal cord of human beings and other mammals can be subdivided into smaller regions according to gross appearance, embryology or cellular organization. At the top a human brain has been drawn so that its internal structures are visible through "transparent" outer layers of the cerebrum. The most general way of dividing the brain is into hindbrain, midbrain and forebrain. The hindbrain includes the cerebellum. The midbrain includes the two elevations known as the inferior and superior colliculi. The forebrain is more complex. Its outer part is the cerebral hemisphere, the surface of which is the convoluted sheet of the cerebral cortex, which incorporates the hippocampus, the neocortex and the olfactory fields. Within the hemisphere are the amygdala and corpus striatum.

neuropeptides, as well as by RNA, neurones, proteins and chemicals as they travel throughout the body.

Hormones actively assist communications between nerves in the bodybrain's somatopsychic system and "thus, the stuff of thought is everywhere", according to Dr. David C. Chamberlain who specializes in psychotherapy on prenatal problems. He points out that neuropeptides form a network between nervous, endocrine and immune systems through receptor sites embedded in each of those three systems. (Chamberlain 1990 [2])

Although recognizing the important role the body's physiochemistry plays in memory and consciousness, Chamberlain falls back on "an immaterial substrate" to explain memory storage. However, though a memory storage system is still not identifiable, there is no need to dump it wholesale into something vague and "immaterial".

This introduces us to the need for a more integrative conceptual view of what goes on between feelings, psychological memory and neurology. We realize now that memories and their attendant feelings are not located in the brain or in any one place, but are the outcome of a process of interactive psychoneurological, unifunctional activities of the bodymind. When a memory occurs in consciousness it usually has many physical, emotional, visual, auditory and verbal components. It draws on all the resources of the body and its organs, physically, chemically, electromagnetically, and neurologically to make its statement.

But, it may be asked, where are the specific receptor, storage and transmission cells receiving the information and moving the data through the nervous system? How is the right place for data recognized? Is a new event "captured" in an existing memory trace by means of neuropeptide receptors which already have some characteristics with which the new event can somehow identify? In the case of completely new learning, such as occurs in children, are perhaps receptors hungrily searching for neuropeptides they can imbibe so as to stabilize themselves into configurations that can become active in the nervous system, and ultimately capture new, appropriate memories? These are questions that can only be partly answered as yet.

Recently, a molecule called protein kinase C (PKC) which operates within the surface membranes of nerve cells has been implicated in triggering cells to store short-term memory. It is a marvelously complicated system whose description is not needed here, involving the absorbtion of calcium and the closing of potassium pores by nerve cells acting in collaboration with other proteins and molecules within the cell to assist in both storage and recall.

Interestingly, it has been found that prenatal rabbits store PKC around the hypothalamus until birth following which PKC enters the hypothalamus and from there travels into nerve cell dendrites to promote the storage of experience needed for survival (Ezzell 1991 [3]). Later, we will examine this extraordinary capability in greater depth for its implications in homeostasis and survival in facilitating learning and memory processes in daily life and in dreamwork.

These bodymind configurations facilitated by PKC in rabbits suggest what may occur on levels of increasing complexity in humans. PKC stored very early in life, perhaps prenatally, may serve as a part of the human storage system for visual, auditory and verbal, etc. events. These events may become triggered or jostled into activity when new, familiar-seeming stimuli enter the system. Whether the jostling will result in repression, memories that lead to dreams, passive or active recall, will depend on many other aspects of the psychoneurological and emotional state of affairs which decide how a person deals with memories. Interestingly, PKC has also been implicated in the development of Alzheimer's disease which is basically a bodymind problem whose symptom is the extensive loss of memory. (See Miller 1993 - *The Psychobiological Nature of Reality with a Theory About Alzheimer's* [4] for an expanded view of how bodymind may create a disease process.)

In endeavoring to synthesize mind and body into a unifunctional activity and to describe how this actually happens, we have already gathered together some research and ideas on the physiological and psychological levels, but have not included the metaphysical level beyond some brief dynamic descriptions of it. This problem will be addressed at various times in greater detail, but for now let it suffice to offer the reader a generalized account of the dynamics of bodymind in preparation for the next chapter on the quontic psychological system.

For a unifunctional system to be effective there must be capabilities of communcation between all its parts. In the quontic system, it will be necessary to look at transmissions of signals limited by the speed of light, and therefore browse in Relativity theory. Basically, we will additionally need to know how information equivalent to memories can undergo transformations from the unseen universe, which we call the fifth dimension, to become converted into communications on the pragmatic level of the third dimension.

It is difficult for scientific persons at times because the bodymind, feelings and memories, like consciousness, are not things in themselves. They are produced through a complex process. They can become emphemeral, become lost or changed or conflict with other persons' views of what happened instead of remaining objective data. Nevertheless, memories as well as feelings serve a purpose which is intimately linked to survival and homeostasis at all levels: psychological, physiological and transpersonal. This means that even daily tasks that we may take for granted (washing our teeth, getting good grades, going to work, having supportive friends and lovers, seeing a psychotherapist or a doctor, joining a religious group, cooking and eating) are different ways we are basically engaged in survival and homeostasis-enhancing activities, for the most part. The possibility and the very shape of such activities, it appears, have developed not simply through habits shaped by parents while growing up, but by the culture as well. Information empowering us to do this is also transmitted through inherited evolutionary processes in DNA.

We have all grown past infancy but we all remain infants to the degree that we all retain memories that nourish us about our survival attachment to our mothers and fathers. And we can remember and repeat activities and continue relationships due to the marvelous capacity for memories and feelings that we have developed as part of our evolutionary heritage. Jung's Archetype Theory states that culture is shaped by such memories (Jung 1964 [5]) (Jaynes 1976 [6]). It's important to examine the system of brain communication and its varied systems in order to understand consciousness, memory and what we have gained from evolution. In doing so, we will take data that is known and organize it into relationships that risk derision from medical and scientific authorities.

Brain as a Communication Process

In Paul McLean's model of the triune brain, the brain stem is the oldest evolutionary part of the system, regulating vital body functions of heartbeat and respiration. Next oldest is the limbic system or rhinencephalon, the communications link between the brainstem and the newest part of the brain, the cerebrum. (Take another look at Figure 8.,*The Brain and Spinal Cord.*)

The limbic system is an organizing center for neurotransmitters that converge together. They translate neurological messages into consciousness which turns it into what we call the awareness of emotions or feelings. At the neurological reception center in the limbic system, it requires the further exchange of bodybrain messages to decide what to do with them. Similarly there are organizing centers throughout the brain for various aspects of bodily functions such as ⁻1ove-ment, olfaction and vision which receive neurotransn. ʳers from the body and send neurochemical transmitters out to other body and brain parts which helps to keep them functioning as a network of interconnected and related parts.

For instance, that part of the brain that manages the function of the throat and voice box organizes these messages from the bodymind into the form of sound we call speech, another part of the brain organizes its messages into music, another into writing and another into dance and so on. Any expressive action we take is the result of how the bodymind uses its messages within the organism, and that is an extraordinarily complicated network of events. We know they become stored because we remember expressive actions that we initiate within ourselves as well as those that affect us whose origin is external to ourselves. But science cannot prove this experimentally. It is discarded as subjective data.

All of this externally and internally induced sensory-motor information passes through the limbic system which includes thalamus and hypothalamus, amygdala, hippocampus, as well as many other parts which are not as significant for this presentation. It's overall job is to maintain the body's state of alertness and emotional balance.

The hippocampus is apparently essential in learning because it converts information from short-term to long-term memory. "It constantly checks information relayed to the brain by the senses and compares it to experience."(Pinchot 1984 [7]) The thalamus is a major relay station passing information from sensory and motor nerves directly to the brain after "analysing" it, therefore, possibly making decisions about what should and should not pass into conscious awareness, acting as a gatekeeper to consciousness.

The hypothalamus is a small cluster of nerve cells from which arise feelings of pleasure, punishment, hunger, thirst, sexual arousal, aggression and rage. And through its connections with the brainstem below, the hypothalamus maintains physiological homeostasis, sensing and sending feedback out about the body's internal temperature, hunger, thirst and equilibrium.

The amygdala, as well as the hippocampus, send messages to the hypothalamus, possibly forwarding impulses and information from lower centers about rage and aggression.

The amygdala also transmits sensory information from the olfactory bulb, more useful in lower animals than in man. It's apparent that all of the activities described for the hypothalamus and amygdala, indeed for the entire limbic system, are crucial for homeostasis and survival.

In addition, all these aspects of the limbic system play a crucial role in feelings and memories. What we "remember" physiologically is the repetition of a pathway that was established by the neurochemical transmitters triggered into action by a psychological stimulus from birth and perhaps prebirth onward, in every part of our body. The initial pathways for remembering were laid down during our developmental years, or even in the womb as Chamberlain, Grof (1985) [8], Miller and other regression and primal oriented therapists believe, and these became channels in which later events reinforced, altered or buried what we can and cannot remember (and feel).

The most critical memories for regression therapies are those of childhood, infancy and birth. The memories of those periods are most sensitive to feeling helpless and dependent on others to manage threats to survival. Of course, if the very persons on whom we are supposed to depend for survival themselves become threats to it, then that is what we remember and defense mechanisms with all their attendant seeds for neurosis, or psychosis, in later life are implanted very early in the bodymind. These are what grow, accumulating reinforcement during the developmental years along with the other experiences accumulated during one's lifetime.

These are also the events so deeply buried in the unconscious they become forgotten. Nevertheless, they continue to motivate daily behavior. Since they can become repressed, defended and made to become inaccessible to the individual, their recall, discharge and integration is what makes psychotherapy necessary and successful. Consciousness is the medium in the therapy process that provides the display screen making processing of these memories possible.

The following is a transcipt of part of a session in the middle of treatment which exemplifies the presence of emotional connections between past and present attitudes and behavior.

Hilda

Hilda came in and sat down on the couch and complained that she felt lethargic, didn't want to do anything. She was tall, naturally attractive without enhancements, large boned and athletic looking. Her husband had left about three years ago and she'd had sporadic, unfulfilling affairs.

Today she had work to do and needed to go out (she worked independently at home) but didn't want to do the work and didn't want to leave the house. Her daughter had been ill a few days so she stayed inside to take care of her and now her daughter was back in school but she didn't want to go out again. She was depressed. This happened to her periodically. It was probably due to the winter weather, she said.

I proposed to her that, if she had nothing else on her mind, this might provide material for a session. She didn't know how it could, but she was willing.

In several minutes (she'd been working with me for about five months and was familiar with my methods) she was talking about feeling like this as a little girl. It was as if she wanted something. She wanted to be cradled or rocked, but it was nonsense because nobody could do that for her, she had to take care of herself. I asked her whether she could tell her mother what she wanted. She couldn't, her mother wouldn't know what to do. Her eyes began to well up with tears. She recalled having many fears as a little girl and how useless it was to tell her mother. She was always very nervous as a child. She was afraid of strange men, afraid that one might be in the house or under the bed, she often had a dream that someone with a knife would attack her in the back of the neck, pictures in dreams would seem to come to life and move about. No one ever did anything, but that was what she was afraid of happening.

I didn't know the cause of these fears but saw many possibilities including birth trauma (generalized survival anxiety), past lives (the pictures coming to life or the man with the knife) a repressed incest experience (basic fear of men).

What happened when she tried to tell her mother about her fears? Her mother would try to tell her it was alright and try to comfort her, but her mother was robot-like and didn't believe it herself. She felt her mother was very fearful too but covered it up. She always slept with her mother in her mother's bed, especially after they moved to another city and her father didn't move with them because they had separated. She found out later that he slept with other women and he was also an alcoholic. He came to visit them but didn't sleep over. In response to my questions she said that the fears actually were strongest after they moved.

I asked whether she could tell her father about these fears. She began to cry more profusely. She didn't want to tell him. Whenever she went to visit him at his house he would insist that she had problems and would try to draw her out, even if she felt happy. She felt very confused about him. She would get angry and tell him she never wanted to see him again, then call a few weeks later. He'd be charming and would talk about himself but he seemed to forget that she was a little girl with a problem and it would drive her crazy to be with him. She hated going to his house but was helpless to change things.

Hilda didn't want to deal with these problems because they were too painful. I suggested that her little girl was still very much alive inside her and still affected her feelings. That seemed to make her cry more. She knew that and that she would probably have to deal with it because it affected her relationships with men, but she hated doing it, she hated spending money on it, she was sick and tired of having problems about her father. Most of the session seemed to be spent crying about what she didn't want to do. Nevertheless, I felt it was productive because she had touched base with her fearfulness as well as with her anger and need under the depression.

Toward the end of the session I asked whether she had gained any insight about the reason for feeling so lethargic. After much avoidance she acknowledged it might be related to her unhappiness as a child, that she was carrying a lot of baggage around with her. It interfered with her relationships with men too because after a year or so of a relationship she would always get into this lethargic state, she said. She wanted the men to do everything for her and became very demanding. It always broke up the relationship. She wanted them to make up for the security, love and caring she never received from either mother or father.

I still harbored many unanswered questions about Hilda's fears but felt that this was about as far as she wanted to go at this point. I simply emphasized the importance of these memories. She said that she had already cried a lot in private but it hadn't done any good. I said that the connections to her feelings were important and that as she continued to discharge them the connections to her present life would become more evident. It would change the way she felt and she would feel less need to cry. But it couldn't all be done in one session. She left therapy about three months later feeling better. I accidently ran into her about a year later and she still felt good and had been working steadily.

Comments

This case clearly demonstrates the protective function of the defense system which limits and blocks accessing feelings and memories, which are "normal" functions of the 3D aspect of consciousness. Reading under the defenses, it seems the lethargy was provoked by her daughter's illness and taking care of her reminded her that she had no one to administer to her needs when she was a child. She didn't want to take care of anyone else, not even of herself and didn't expect anyone to want to take care of her, but was not aware of her unsatisfied need and the anger around it or how it damaged her life. From prior sessions, I knew that this woman had access to 5D energies, but the defense system was very powerful on this day. Undoubtedly her lethargy was real and physical but the reason for its presence was emotional and tied to her history.

We have already examined and will continue to search for the interrelationships between the physiological and psychological components of the bodymind. What we have found, to some degree constituting the structure of consciousness, are paths built up by our neurologically-developed and neurochemically-maintained pathways, as described in the chapter called "Models of Consciousness". These respond actively when they are triggered by psychological patterns of stimuli. Neither long nor short term memories can be said to reside solely in the brain, nor solely in the mind, because the neurochemical process and neural pathways involved cover the unifunctional bodymind, in all its dynamics.

Transformational Dynamics

Further research findings enable us to link biological dynamics with psychodynamics. Over the years, since 1893 and the early theories of Santiago Ramon Y Cajal [9], much neurobiological work has been done on the biochemistry of memory. Such research now indicates that signals entering the body through two or more sensory modalities simultaneously will link up with their neural pathways interconnected through biochemical transmitter and recepter chemicals. Cells in the hippocampus rich in a molecule called the NMDA receptor molecule (N-methyl D-asparte) can turn on the biochemical reactions that lead to encoding memories. This receptor molecule, it has been found, is important not only for encoding memories but for developmental learning processes as well by creating new circuitry, especially in the infant brain. (Johnson 1988 [10])

A memory process starts, according to current research, when sensory messages stimulate the cells of the brain. Then a neurotransmitter molecule is released by a neuron in the brain into the synapse between itself and another neuron. Receptor channels are opened up in the receptor neuron, letting potassium and sodium ions into the cells. When these charged ions accumulate, channels sensitive to voltage charges are also tripped open bringing electromagnetic discharges into play. When ions flood into the neuron they cause it to fire which in turn sends a signal down the line into the next neuron. Connecting neurons then develop a lasting circuitry which is sensitive to transmitters and receptors travelling from the sensory equipment to the brain (and probably other appropriate parts of the body as well). Such circuitry's ability to store memories also depends upon the accumulation of sufficient strength in the synaptic connections. High frequency bursts of electricity indeed were found to stimulate neural pathways in the hippocampus sufficiently to reliably enhance the responsivity of such electrical circuits. According to many scientists, this biochemical and electrical stimulation and response in neural pathways is what must be happening when a memory is recorded.

More than that, the introduction of high-frequency bursts of electrical charges, it was found, could turn up the volume controls in the synapses so that circuits would respond more vigorously to stimulation. This is important in order to record memory and, I would add, it is probably also vital to memory as a responsive circuit, during the recall of memories.

Theta Rhythm, Memory and Evolution

There is additional relevant neurological research on the nature of memories which has to do with their relationship to survival, and ultimately to evolution. It has to do with the involvement of a slow brain wave frequency called the Theta rhythm and its related electrical and biochemical interactions. This is very important for the quontic psychological system because Theta rhythm offers a third dimensional key into the quontic loop and therefore into the electromagnetic field in the fifth dimension. It has been found to have a significant effect upon learning in daily life, in meditation and in the REM phase of sleep. Active during stimuli involving survival, it is a significant part of the homeostatic system involving memory and evolution.

Researches show that Theta rhythm is the electrical level of brainwave activity that is prevalent during deep meditation, daily learning and deep sleep. It has been found that the Theta level is accessed biochemically by the NMDA receptor molecule when it is stimulated first by a voltage change and then by a transmitter (glutamate). There are two phases involved, the first preparing the receptor to respond and the second the firing of calcium into the cell which opens the switches for theta activity. A very specific sequence of firings, 10 pairs of 200 millisecond firings occurring every five seconds results in a frequency corresponding to the theta rhythm. On the opposite end, excessive calcium released into neuronal synapses is believed to trigger seizures and brain damage through overstimulation of NMDA receptors. There are additional factors that turn sensitivity up or down based on subtler interactions with other chemicals (such as glycine, an amino acid). (See next page, Figure 9., *Brain-Body Circuitry in Memory Storage*, showing how neural pathways arising from both external and internal stimuli enter the hippocampus where innervations are processed before going into physical and psychological aspects of memory storage.)

During Theta rhythm, according to indications from neurobiological research, is an excellent time for the best learning to occur, and indeed research done many years ago on the relationship between meditation and learning found a strong relationship to be present. It was this relationship that first attracted researchers to study it. Theta is, in effect, the rhythm in which memories are effectively stored, not only becoming activated during meditation but in daily activities as well.

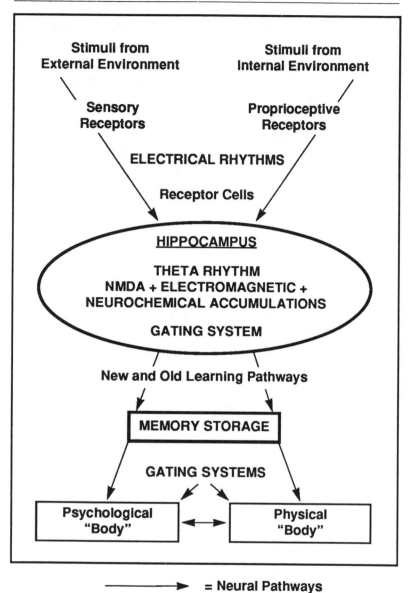

= Neural Pathways

Figure 9.
Brain-Body Circuitry in Memory Storage

Neural pathways arise from both external and internal stimuli and enter the hippocampus where innervations are processed.

Learning and memory storage are so critical for what goes on in daily life that if it is the major factor in learning and storage Theta must be working much more mundanely than was at first thought. (Recall the work in storage and recall performed by PKC with rabbits as subjects, described earlier, in which activities bearing on survival were placed in memory during birth and even perhaps prebirth).

Most recently, it is proposed that during the REM (rapid eye movement) phase of sleep when dreaming occurs, theta rhythm is instrumental in organizing the day's events into a memory storage process. Says Jonathan Winson, Research Professor in Neuroscience at Rockefeller University in New York:

> "Studies of the hippocampus (the brain structure crucial to memory), of rapid eye movement sleep and of a brain wave called theta rhythm suggest that dreaming reflects a pivotal aspect of the processing of memory....They appear to be the nightly record of a basic mammalian memory process: the means by which animals form strategies for survival and evaluate current experience in light of those strategies." (Winson 1990 [11])

Subprimate animals awakened during REM sleep get up ready to attack or defend even though immediate danger is not present, obviously in response to dreams in which survival activities are being integrated. This response is not available when theta is not being recorded. Sensory stimuli travelling between the neocortex (the newest part of the cortex), the limbic system and the brainstem where theta appears to originate, together form the core of the memory system in the brain, according to Winson. So many receptor sites for neuropeptides have also been found in the brainstem that it is evident that neuropeptides also play a significant role in the limbic system, in memory and probably in dreaming.

Out of the above, a picture is developing of the biological details that enable us to fill out the neurological sketch drawn earlier with the work of E.R. John. Theta rhythm is a survival-sensitive brain wave which is also implicated in feeling and memories connected with survival. We have already seen that neuropeptides operating between the brainstem and the neocortex also have a fundamental role in the recording of memories. It is possible that this network is a key to the access of experiences such as the case histories presented in these chapters.

It is very interesting that theta rhythm has also been found active during meditative states. Does this give us a clue that ties it into recall of fifth dimensional information? Failures in access to meditation and fifth dimensional consciousness might be due to failure to activate theta rhythm in the subject.

Winson's neurological research is pivotal for understanding the brain's aspect of the relationships between memory, survival, evolution and homeostasis, and ultimately the physiological component in the development of consciousness. He clarifies how the hippocampus, rapid eye movement (REM) sleep, dreams, and theta rhythm are all crucial to memory.

"They [dreams] appear to be the nightly record of a basic mammalian memory process: the means by which animals [as well as humans] form strategies for survival and evaluate current experience in light of those strategies".

Thus, for instance, Hilda's rejection of her father and her initial refusal to communicate with him had become a way of insuring her survival in regard to his traumatic effect upon her. Rejection of parents following cases of childhood trauma as well as holding onto them, are usually survival motivated. However, repression of the traumatic events themselves by defense mechanisms and attendant inability to recall associated feelings constitutes a core problem for psychotherapy because recall is catharctic and healing. Is theta rhythm also blocked by defense mechanisms?

Theta rhythm appears in the hippocampus of animals during awake as well as sleeping hours when there is sur-

vival-specific activity such as exploration in the rat, preda-
tory behavior in the cat, etc. The hippocampus is also
involved in memory processing and it may therefore be true
that dreaming is the way the animal processes daily survival
activities into memory.

Following the trail of neurological research regarding
memory shows us that the hippocampus is a receiving,
storage and retransmission area for Long Term Potentiation,
as long term memory reception and storage is called. The
NMDA receptor molecule has sites embedded in the hippocampus and in neurons throughout the new brain or neocortex. Theta rhythm, it turns out, activates NMDA receptors
in the hippocampus. Furthermore, LTP (long term potentiation), intrinsic to the memory process, is dependent on theta
rhythm signals and is absent when theta is not present.
Thus, theta rhythm and NMDA appear to have an important
hand in releasing long term memories, therefore in homeostasis and survival.

Sensory information, which follows a neuronal path into
the hippocampus becomes partitioned into 200-millisecond
'bites' by theta rhythm, allowing for storage and LTP. During
sleep, it was found by Winson and his colleagues, the same
neurones that were fired by theta rhythm while awake
(during survival related activity) "fired at a significantly
higher rate than their previous sleeping baseline", suggesting reinforcement during sleep of information encoded while
awake.

Furthermore, Winson says, "Evidence that theta rhythm
encodes memories during REM sleep may be derived not only
from neuro-scientific studies but also from evolution." Though
theta rhythm appears to be present in mammals called
echidna during daytime foraging for food, the echidna do not
have REM sleep but have prefrontal lobes that are even
relatively larger than that of human beings. Evolution
apparently devised an economic solution for expanding its
memory storage further by connecting theta rhythm with a
REM sleep stage during which memory for survival activities
could be integrated and reinforced.

For Quontic Psychology, this is a perfect example of the operation of the homeostatic principle. Without having to further expand the prefrontal cortex, which would make the head become too heavy to sustain upright body balance, a way was developed for survival to be enhanced through the brain's available memory mechanisms by the development of REM sleep. It remains primarily visual in operation, much as it was and still is in marsupial animals, prior to the evolutionary development of placental animals and homo sapiens, as suggested by differences in brain anatomy between echidna, marsupials and placentals. With less prefrontal area required to process and store information, the brain could shrink in size and focus greater attention on refined perceptual and cognitive functions in higher species.

"Consistent with evolution and evidence derived from neuroscience and reports of dreams, I suggest that dreams reflect an individual's strategy for survival", states Winson. Dreams remain in the core of the unconscious, at which level they are primarily sensory and visual, until triggered into consciousness either by some association or an attempt to recall their content. That content is fundamentally intensely emotional because fears, insecurities, needs, etc. that affect survival are their substance. Most intense psychotherapy experiences have this common source in survival anxiety. Additional experimental research work reveals that tracing associations backward returns the content toward early childhood, birth and pre-birth experiences during which survival was invariably fragile or severely threatened.

There is no more crucial event for the survival of the individual than his birth. Birth primals are seldom peaceful and are memories of felt threats to survival which appear to remain in their pristine form when they return from the unconscious during a birth primal in the psychotherapy process. Hard though it is to believe (since scientific method is not applicable to reliving a birth experience - and does that mean we are not born if science cannot replicate the event of our birth experimentally?), patients do recall with vivid feelings what it is like to be lacking oxygen either due to the mother's constricted air intake or having the umbilical cord wrapped around the foetus, trapped in a birth canal that is too small for a little human body, or panicked due to sensitivity to a mother's volatile emotional state. Sometimes there is a memory of an attempted abortion, being rejected during foetal development, or depression on the part of the mother which was not shared verbally until the adult confronted the parent with this knowledge, at which time it was more often than not confirmed.

These early memories of the fight for survival remain embedded in the nervous system as somatopsychological memories, perhaps in the young hippocampus. They absorb later events into their psychoneurological content to become a network of emotions and activities that affect daily life as well as dreams. The core of these dream-based emotions that motivate a variety of stressful and sometimes unrealistic daily activities might be the threat to survival that is psycho-neurologically imbedded during birth. As will be indicated later, survival is also the core of the process that motivates psychological interaction with physiological evolutionary changes even while it helps determine the content of dreams. Patients who relive those primal birth memories discharge their emotional content as much as possible, thereby opening up space in their character structure for a different, more positive and more effective self-concept, based on a reduced threat to survival. Releasing the psychophysiological effects of the memory alters their psychophysiological state.

In order to trace some of these relationships within the physiological organism, see the next page and Figure 10., *The Inheritance Pathway*, showing the pathways through which the DNA of genetic inheritance is processed in the neuroanatomy to meet the effects of behavioral learning about survival in memories and dreams.

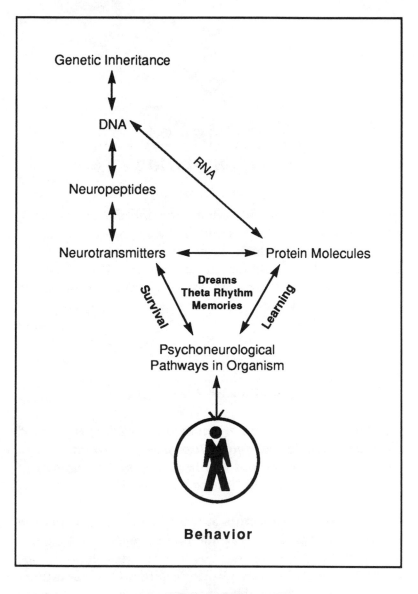

Figure 10.
The Inheritance Pathway,

showing the pathways through which the DNA of genetic inheritance is processed in the neuroanatomy to meet the effects of behavioral learning.

The Quontic System: Transmutations

"Are not gross Bodies and Light convertible into one another, and may not Bodies receive much of their Activity from the Particles of Light which enter their Composition?....The changing of Bodies into Light and Light into Bodies, is very conformable to the Course of Nature, which seems delighted with Transmutations."

— Isaac Newton

The Meaning of Fragmentation

Quontic Psychology is an example of a system of integrated physical, psychological and metaphysical interrelationships which seeks to relate and organize the psychodynamics of matter and mind into an integrated science.

One of the central points of Quontic Psychology and the unifunctional mind is that a homeostatic energy principle is a basic driving force in the universe, not just in ourselves, which makes the universe work despite its fragmentation. Homeostatic energy enables events to swing along a certain degree of arc like a pendulum going from Yin to Yang, piercing through and unifying the fragments in the course of the total arc of its swing. Most of us don't have the breath of vision to see and unify the swing through more than several fragments of arc at a time and some of us grasp more than others. However, developing a perception that does unify the fragments of existence is natural for some and can be learned by others. Eastern practices were developed specifically for the purpose of teaching us how to unify the fragmentation. Psychotherapy, if effective, does it as well. (See Figure 2. — *Synchronistic Perception in a Fragmented State* — on page xiv.)

The quotation by Newton on the previous page is one of those statements that cuts through to the whole of life simultaneously. It can be read as the relationship of light and mass to one another anticipating in effect Einstein's energy formula $E=MC^2$, or as the relationship of spirit (light) to matter (mass), therefore, transposing terms again, of fifth to third dimensional phenomena. It's rather strange that both Newton and Einstein believed in God but that neither attempted to relate their theories to more than a material universe. It would be an incredibly bold stroke to find a mathematical method to relate Einstein's energy formula to the transformation or the communication of spirit and matter. (It would state that energy is equal to mass times the speed of the influx of spirit, squared. Something about that rings intuitively true.) For the present, however, we will have to be satisfied with a less dramatic description of the universe.

Now imagine that the swing of the pendulum in Figure 2 not only traverses the 180 degree arc from left to right under a horizontal line, but that it also swings upward above the horizontal, invisibly, in a mirror image arc, synchronistically with the visible arc below the horizontal. The second arc is a metaphor representing the spiritual and paranormal domain. Together they form a perception of reality that is synchronized by the continuous flow between the arcs, like our intuitive interpretation of $E=MC^2$.

There are ordinarily two common, generally unsatisfying ways in which people attempt to deal with the totality of experience, represented by the two halves of the circle.

One way is to deny the existence of anything not palpable to rigorous intellectual, materialistic, scientific knowledge and experiment, (relying solely on the lower half of the circle) making the upper half undeserving of recognition in reality. The other way is to turn the picture upside down and call the invisible, spiritual, non-material upper half of the arc the total reality, denying the significance of empirical reality and calling it irrelevant as if it were invisible, thereby again losing the unifunctional relationship between the lower and the upper halves.

In Eastern philosophy, a few Yogis, not the majority, have attempted the second feat by denying the relevance of the material world within a total picture of reality. They have made the same mistake as the materialists who rejected the spiritual part of the arc. Novices, entranced by the mystery of the transcendental experience, some of whom find it too painful to deal with three dimensional reality, commit the same kind of existential error. These people believe that focussing on spiritual love, or past lives, or spirit entities, for example, will solve all the problems that exist for themselves and humanity as well. It doesn't work that way because although the two levels interact and affect one another, each has its own rules of operation which must be understood and attended to if changes are to be made.

Of course, I am pointing out the extremes. Most people, and the most astute gurus, understand that the true state of affairs resides in the swing of the pendulum within the totality of its two arcs, making a complete circle. Jesus, Moses and Buddha, within their very different conceptualizations that evolved into major religions, did understand this and fought great personal battles within themselves and with their environments to bring the two into balance, implicitly to create a better homeostasis for people than existed in their time.

It is common in our society to block out the top half of the arc entirely, reject, deny or disown it, and regard materialism as the totality of experience. We are, in Western society, personally, socially and environmentally now paying the price for such an empirically limited view of life. Politicians, like scientists, are vulnerable to this mistake because politics, like science, depends solely on pragmatic techniques and outcomes for its measurement of success.

Empirical physicists, propelled by a holistic, homeostatic drive of their own are looking for the Grand Unified Theory behind their fragmented physics. My guess is that they won't find it until they discover a way to rationalize their empirical, scientific logic to include either God, or Consciousness, or Infinte Self-Energy, or Homeostasis, or the equivalent thereof in their GUTs (to be read organically, in addition to Grand Unified Theory). They are looking for the right thing in the wrong way by being unwilling to expand the traditional scientific, experimental paradigm into the upper arc.

They are looking in the particle for the unification-God, and they are dismayed they haven't found Him yet. However, their paradigm masks or rejects the evidence so they can't see it. They have already found the desired unification concepts but have not been able to recognize them. They haven't been able to stretch their perceptions to reconcile their findings about concepts that include infinite states of mass and energy within their materialism because infinity, like states beyond the speed of light, can't be descriptively conceptualized, or measured. Infinity is represented by a symbol for what it is but cannot be described beyond the symbol. What scientists still don't know will still fill many volumes of experimental literature even though they periodically announce that they have reached the end of the road, know all about reality, and that there is nothing unknown left for science to discover. Who was it that said that acknowledgement of ignorance is the beginning of wisdom?

We will explore, in the chapter called "The Purple Cow", the many ways they have found and denied the reality of the upper half of the arc. In that chapter we will find that they have discovered infinite quantities in their equations (which prevented them from confining their concepts to a strictly finite materialistic mathematical position in evaluating data) and then rejected it, as well as other "anomalies" that become explanations for quontic psychology, as we shall see in the next couple of chapters.

Dealing with and manipulating infinite and negative numbers, and energy that appears to come from less than zero mass, continually reappears in mathematical equations. To accept such concepts destroys the illusion for physicists that the universe begins at some empirical, measurable, finite point greater than Zero. From our perspective it could be said that the empirical design of fragmentation and frag- mented consciousness begin at a point greater than zero and the Uncreated Whole exists at a point below zero mass and energy. There is no way to measure an Uncreated Whole because it exists prior to fragmentation and therefore prior to material creation and mathematics. The Uncreated Whole might be described as a state of unboundaried consciousness, following the Eastern paradigm. In Western religions, that state of paradise, God's domain, existed first and gave rise to fragmented, materialistic reality (symbolically Adam bit- ing into the apple—the temptation of knowledge giving rise to the sin of materialistic consciousness which fragmented him from the uncreated whole of consciousness, and particu- larly dividing love into male and female forms). Nevertheless, we know through our religious and cultural mythology that our fragmented, boundaried existence above zero mass still reflects and manifests the presence of unboundaried con- sciousness which is wholeness and is its source.

In this respect I would like to quote an anecdote from Richard Feynman's Physics Nobel Prize award acceptance address. In it, he discusses the difficulty of keeping track of all the active variables which occur in an electron particle's past and present behavior. Attempting to keep track of the electron's erratic course makes it confoundingly difficult for the physicist to know all the active variables that will affect a particle's future position and can reduce his work to book- keeping. This is made worse since all electrons have the same charge and the same mass.

Feynman recalls, "...I received a telephone call one day at the graduate college at Princeton from Professor Wheeler, in which he said, 'Feynman, I know why all electrons have the same charge and the same mass.' 'Why?', Feynman asked. He was told by Wheeler, 'Because, they are all the same electron!'"

All electrons are one electron. Fragmentation manifests its source in unity. God made man (many men and women, fragmentation) in his own image (oneness, the unfragmented whole). Chaos turns to order when underlying patterns are revealed. Every component in the image of a hologram contains the entire image. When man submits to the emptiness that is wholeness he unifies the fragmentation in his Being. He gives up Maya, the great illusion of material reality, and joins the Godhead in Nirvana. How many ways does it need to be said?

Yet, Wheeler, for example, states he is completely opposed to anything with paranormal or spiritual concepts in it and calls such ideas pseudo-science. Heinz Pagels, the deceased former president of the New York Academy of Sciences sent me a note in response to my question, stating I might use his ideas regarding complexity in my writing, but that he did not believe in the existence of paranormal phenomena. Nevertheless, "all is one" is an ultimate "fact of life" in Eastern mysticism and in holistic consciousness just as it is for the electron and for physicists seeking the ultimate GUT. The Grand Unified Theory is the All Is One of quantum physics. It is unfortunate that Wheeler, following his communication to Feynman, could not reconcile his scientific method with that of his spontaneous spiritual-scientific insight.

In part, I see a job begging to get done, as do many other writers in the areas of science and metaphysics, in bringing these two antagonistic studies of science and religion together. Resolution is needed because the antagonism exists within the individual as strongly as within society.

The spiritual dimension, which existed in humankind's awareness at least five thousand years before scientific method came into being, has the edge. Science is like a son who is too afraid of being too close to his father because, even though he has a strong unconcious identity with him, he is afraid that if he succombs to the wisdom of the father (intuitive spiritual knowledge), he will be swallowed up and lose his hard-won separate identity, which to him becomes all of reality.

Even though they are saying the same things very often, the younger one has to continue to protest and rebel and declaim his difference from the parent, as an affirmation of the separation and fragmentation. There is no doubt, in thus asserting his individual strength, he discovers new things that are important and useful to himself and society. But, he needs time to develop security in his own sense of individuality. Paradoxically, not until a person feels secure enough in his individuality can the growing child within begin to release himself from the conflict with the parent and attain peace in being who he is and affirm his, as well as his parents', divinity.

Finally, giving up the problems of striving for individuality (by knowing that he has it) enables a person to accept the basic holistic, spiritual and homeostatic energy state in which the universe fundamentally thrives because then only can it provide fundamental nourishment and continuity. In this way a person attains a Real Self and a Real Ego-awareness. The motivation for further striving then becomes to attain mastery as much as possible of one's inner potential capabilities—increasing self-awareness and well-being by healing the internal split from unboundaried wholeness. The framework of values then becomes much larger than egoism or individuality. Then one can rejoin a wholistic consciousness on the larger scale and rediscover the Harmonic Self. Perhaps it is possible to translate Buddahood into Western terms after all.

In a significant way, integration begins when we commit ourselves to engage in releasing ourselves from the state of fragmentation in the lower half of the arc. It is a gradual development and not a sudden miracle. It opens gradually with acceptance of the currents of spiritual awareness and self-knowledge that are continually at work between fifth and third dimensional states of being.

In its fragmented state, energy is held back by numerous blockages. Engaging in the process of contacting psychic, emotional and physical wholeness, formerly blocked energy can be released to flow toward the arc's upper half and become the crucible for further growth toward self-actualization. The split of the circle into two halves disappears when energy flows between them. This may happen periodically, offering a sense of total well-being, until the fragmentation of material life takes over again. Thus we lose Paradise many times in one lifetime while expanding our connection and our knowledge of it.

Quontic Psychology attempts to understand this problem in human as well as in scientific terms. Human consciousness, flowing between the two halves when its energy is unblocked, provides a key through self-awareness to the integration of the two halves within a psychophysiological context.

However, dealing with fragmentation and releasing energy from blocked states cannot be done without risk-taking of a kind from which people tend to retreat. Accepting risks provides the rewarding outcome of an increase in capacity for awareness on levels of mind, body, feeling and spirit which heightens one's appreciation for the beautiful possibilities of the life in oneself and in others. Underneath it all, unblocking is healing, growth is healing, change is healing, and trusting our own powers is most of all fulfilling as well as healing.

The following model is based on the need to solve a problem of the relationship between two kinds of experience, both of which appear to me to be vital and true sources of energy and motivation in human functioning. It is partially based on scientific research, as well as on metaphysical, anecdotal and intuitive sources of information, as evident from the foregoing and following chapters. In fact, the beginning of the following description may appear so metaphysical as to be out of place with the rest of these chapters

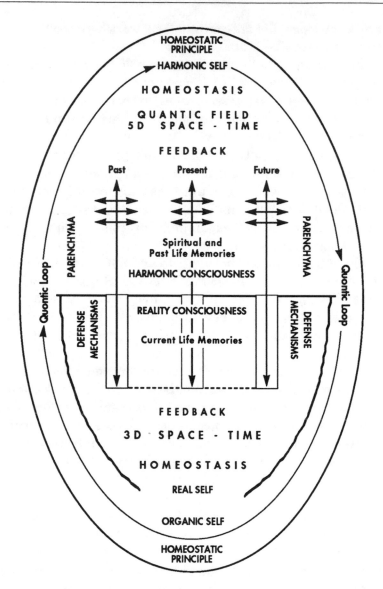

Figure 11.
Quontic Psychology,

a systematic look at the ideas that are used consistently
throughout this book.

which are scientifically oriented. However, the metaphysical ideas are common currency for what later becomes translated into psychological and scientific language. It is simultaneously intuitive, logical, irrational, speculative, and integrative. I simply wish to add that it is not necessary to believe that everything in it is true, but I hope it does show that there is value in attempting the integration.

We are ready to look systematically at the ideas that describe Quontic Psychology. Refer to the diagram on the previous page, Figure 11., *Quontic Psychology*, a systematic look at the ideas that are used consistently throughout this book.

Studying the "Glossary of Terms..." at the end of the chapter will further promote comprehension of the system.

Special Role of the Quontic Warehouse

In the quontic psychological system I have divided memory and its role in consciousness into two halves, for the sake of clarity. These two halves are an expansion of the previous diagram on synchronistic perception. It can be understood as describing bi-dimensional aspects of memory and personality . The lower part of the "egg of consciousness" is the commonplace three dimensional level of life as it is lived in the here and now with its effects on consciousness through memories stored within the human body. The upper half is that which exists on the harmonic or fifth dimensional level, having interactions and significant effects on the three dimensional part, yet following different rules of existence (Cipra 1993[1]). Each level has a system that is independent and interactional with the other allowing for simultaneously independent and interactional memory storage and feedback for recall, growth, change and homeostasis. Energy exchange is more or less intensely continuously active between them, perhaps especially visible during REM sleep and during Theta wave activity, as we have seen.

In the upper level fifth dimensional field there is a capacity to contain all that ever was, is and will be which constitutes the content of the quontic warehouse. It is accessible through the quontic loop and if the means of access are available it can provide knowledge about every aspect of life to oneself. In some respects, it is similar to the Akasic Record, which is a similar notion about the storage of all past lives that were ever experienced, but there are profound differences. That difference is the outcome not only of the way the fifth dimension is structured in quontic psychology in having its own paranormal, acausal, non-linear characteristics, but is due to having interactions which create responses to events on the three-dimensional level, understood in everyday terms through experiential, synchronistic, scientific, creative and intuitive ideas.

The information in the quontic warehouse is not static. It is dynamic and changes in response to events occurring on the three-dimensional level. It receives input through feedback from its own as well as from the lower reality level continually and is fluid enough to allow its own information base to be altered by 3D events. In this way it becomes an essential source of alterable, responsive data in a feedback system, with its display and manifestation components participating fully on the functional level of human consciousness.

Special Role of the Quontic Loop

Information in the quontic field and in the quontic warehouse can be accessed within the range of dynamics available in the quontic loop. The quontic field and it's information is a system which is always looking for an opportunity to communicate with the display level in three dimensional reality and may sometimes flood that level of consciousness when it finds itself possible sources of manifestation in particular people. Each manifestation travels an energy circuit with its own peculiar oscillatory frequency between third and fifth dimensions, completing its circle within the quontic loop, manifesting as a thought or image to those people.

Entering consciousness by means of the quontic loop opens up the possibility of channeling to communicate intentionally and instantaneously within its parameters. To use it, one needs to be open to the connection with the energy state that tunes into potentially emergent energies of the display system native to consciousness.

Manifestation of contents of the fifth dimension through spontaneous three-dimensional events are particularly interesting because they are the kind of events sometimes called miracles, such as Joan of Arc's visions that led to her saving France from its enemies, sometimes manifested through gurus and religious leaders, such as the inspiration that enabled Christ and Buddha to understand the relationship between spiritual and daily life and reach the masses with their message, in their own different ways. Spontaneous events may occur in people's everyday lives, sometimes with recognition and sometimes without it, such as the precognition of the death of a loved one without thinking of oneself as a channel. When it does happen, it can result in fear, insecurity and withdrawal if it is not understood and accepted by the person who is manifesting such consciousness.

In the opposite direction, a response of ill-considered "belief" may allow irresponsible or fictitious ego-motivated "evidence" of fifth dimensional manifestation to be taken for an actual manifestation. Differentiation is necessary and valuable on the three dimensional level of reality.

Intentional manifestation, accessed by means of cumulatively higher levels of consciousness, is most highly developed in its human form. The intention to access the fifth dimension through consciousness may very well be the most important of several qualities which differentiated mankind, through evolutionary processes, from lower and earlier forms of life. However, organic evolutionary processes may still be working through other forms of life on this or other planets to produce intentional manifestation, within the constraints of that planet's material and ecological potential. Even on the planet Earth there appear to be forms of consciousness, for example in the case of dolphins, which seem to be close to human consciousness, suggesting conscious evolution may be continuing at the present time in life forms in the ocean as well as on land.

The Parenchyma

Energizing the everyday homeostasis of the universe is the job of what in the quontic system, is called "the Parenchyma". It is not an object but is an organic, naturally homeostatic energy process which, like a huge breath, pulsates outward to send out energy and pulsates inward to absorb energy at rates faster than the speed of light. In physical terms, it is an oscillation or vibration not measureable in three-dimensional terms. Nevertheless, it provides access and outlet to the quontic warehouse in an energy form.

"Inspire" is an interesting word because it retains two meanings not obviously connected, which are actually two sides of the parenchymatic coin. On the one side it means to breathe in air which is essentially molecular energy (H_2O) and on the other side it means to let in and to animate thoughts and feelings that are spontaneously informative and a source of creative activity which is the manifestation of the energy (divine spirit?) animating organic life. The two sides of "inspire" obviously occur in tandem, especially in mysticism. In Hinduism the breath is conceived containing these qualities - the breath is the inhalation and exhalation of the spirit of life.

The opposite of inspire is "expire" meaning out of breath as well as breathing out, which is what happens when we die and we can no longer inspire to remain physically engaged with the parenchyma through active physical consciousness. A three dimensional level of consciousness is then no longer available since the channel of manifestation can no longer inspire (breathe air or life into) itself. Its manifestation must therefore return to a more generic level of function which we call death. However, what little we do know despite the limitations inherent in the structural design of our three dimensional existence indicates that inspiration continues in another way within the fifth dimensional dynamics of parenchymatic and harmonic consciousness.

Harmonic Consciousness

The highest level that we can describe in the quontic field is called the Harmonic Self, though this doesn't mean it is the highest that can exist. It is simply that our form of description of the communications occurring with the tuning-in process available to consciousness does not exceed what we can call the Harmonic Self. It can only be accessed by Harmonic Consciousness which is a means of accessing or tuning in to the most basic, highest levels of unmanifested existence possible. The Harmonic Self is knowable through Harmonic Consciousness by means of levels which have probably been achieved by great religious leaders like Jesus and Buddha, Eastern mystics, yogis and perhaps more recently by Western healers.

Generally then, for everyone, there are channels in consciousness running between the reality and the harmonic levels that provide more or less direct routes of access to the quontic warehouse and to the parenchyma through the quontic loop. Sometimes the evidence for it is as simple as picking up the phone before it rings to call someone who is already on the other end. At other times it may be a psychic healing process in which one trains in healing oneself, as has been done in cancer and other diseases, using imagery and opening accessability channels to healing (parenchymatic/homeostatic) energy.

Access channels can be described empirically by means of technical terms in electromagnetic systems such as resonance, wave frequency, oscillations and the like, but that and the technical aspect of what follows will be left for later.

Channels are energy pathways that exist within the quontic loop. Energy channels vary in their characteristics and are differentiable in electromagnetic dynamics because each channel maintains a different resonance capacity. Synchronous resonance capabilities connecting three dimensional and fifth dimensional kinds of structures allow communications to travel in the appropriate channel between reality and harmonic consciousness within the quontic loop.

In general, what we can do is develop the capability to "tune in" on the reality level to an appropriate "channel" of the feedback system going into the quontic level, its warehouse of memories and its parenchyma, through harmonic consciousness. In the case of humans, tuning in to the quontic level happens intentionally and most dramatically through meditation, channeling, and past life regression, for instance, and it occurs spontaneously in "miracles", near-death, out of body experiences, precognition, and in dreams. Much has been written on the varieties of psychic experience, any of which may be accessed through an appropriately resonant tuning-in process within the quontic loop. This will be described further in later chapters in Part II.

Tuning-In to Consciousness

Consciousness, in order to display its contents, relies on the physical organism, somewhat like the monitor relies on the VCR, or the loudspeakers on the receiver which in turn receive transmissions from the broadcasting studio. Images, words, music and actions are sensory-motor modalities which are translated into consciousness for the reception, transformation and transmission of messages.

Awareness is a product of the feedback system employed by consciousness. It takes and processes information from the body and the environment, from both three dimensional and fifth dimensional sources. Awareness allows a growing sensitivity to what is going on within the basic nature of the person, reflecting itself on the screen of consciousness. There is obviously a processing methodology which sorts out the information which will be displayed, and rejects that which will not be able to make its way through the selection gates (Eccles 1985 [2]).

Gates from the unconscious to the conscious may take different forms. They can be like turnstiles requiring the right kind of coins, but sometimes it is possible to jump over the turnstile to enter; or more sensitively, it may be like tuning in through a wavelength and channel system as on a TV or more complexly yet like a computer, in which it is necessary to open a series of electronic devices in order to enter.

Even more so than the computer, the psychophysiological apparatus has numerous kinds of devices which go into operation prior to a manifestation of information on the consciousness display screen. In psychological terms, there are the defense mechanisms which process information for its acceptability (an acceptable coin) before it will pass information through the gate (for example, from an unconscious or harmonic to a conscious state).

The human organism is both versatile and flexible, therefore, defense mechanisms are not designed with an altogether foolproof set of safeguards. Because it is not foolproof, defense mechanisms and the physiological gates can sometimes be manipulated cleverly by new instruments and methods developed by those people searching for means to display information. If it is in the interests of perceived homeostasis, the new output in consciousness may become integrated into an alteration in the defense system, changing illness into wellness.

Sometimes unintentionally, despite safeguards that our consciously reality-oriented minds set up against displaying the secret domain of the unconscious, triggers will trip it into revealing itself. Paranormal experiences may sometimes happen which are unpremeditated and therefore not anticipated, against which defenses are not yet strong enough or are in the process of breaking down. At other times, the desire to retrieve and display fifth dimensional information is consciously very strong and can be acted upon purposefully and successfully, as in transformative psychotherapy, meditation, remote viewing and channeling experiences, for example. However, at other times, a person consciously wishes to enter the quontic field but unconscious resistances and fears are even more powerful than the conscious intention and the access gates remain closed.

An analogy to the display of information which was intentional but not predictable in content can be made with the following kind of situation in meditation, which I recently experienced. Imagine the following situation.

There is a lighted candle on a small table in front of the meditator (myself in this case) and a small picture of the Buddha, also seated in meditation is positioned behind the candle. The "reality" of my situation takes in all the three dimensional objects present in my frame of reference, myself meditating, the table, the lighted candle, and Buddha sitting in a meditation posture in the picture behind the candle. In a little while, the candle takes on a characteristic that transcends the three dimensional reality and becomes "luminous" in the way that I see it in my mind, and the Buddha looks real and seems full of energy. I haven't lost the "reality" that the Buddha is just a picture, but I allow my consciousness to alter what it is perceiving. It feels like a manifestation of a live Buddha. My feeling is one of surprise, perhaps a little fear. After awhile the image fades.

What happened in my consciousness was that the space between the candle and the Buddha became an alive, energy charged three dimensional area, feeling just the same as the space between myself and the candle. The candle, or "consciousness" had now become a meeting point for us. The display of harmonic consciousness had altered the characteristics of the space, at least temporarily. The effect of "Buddha consciousness" joined my here-and-now consciousness by displaying an expanded reality to me. I felt as if the Buddha was communicating something to me: that our spirits were interchangeable as if I could somehow tune into his spiritual channel. Nothing more than that happened, but it shook me up and I felt profoundly moved.

The display on the screen of my consciousness had received an input from transcendental consciousness to expand the usual display perceived through my senses. The framework of the display still occurred within the usual three dimensions in the context of my body-brain functions, but the usual input displayed on the screen of my consciousness had been expanded to include the additional dimension of the spiritually alive Buddha. A gate had been opened. I have been meditating and studying Buddhist practices for many years or this would not have occurred. This preparatory work had attuned

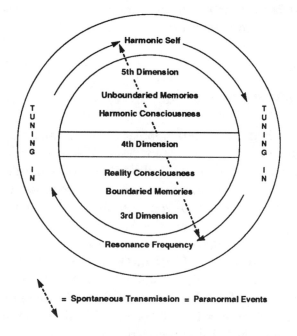

Figure 12.
Memory Retrieval in the Quontic Loop,

displaying paths encompassed by the tuning-process as it signals memories resonant in the 5th and 3rd dimensions.

me to a particular resonance channel which prepared that gate and gave me the needed coin to open it.

(See Figure 12., *Memory in the Quontic Loop*, which displays the paths encompassed by the tuning-process as it signals memories resonant in the 5th and 3rd dimensions. A resonant frequency may be signalled through a purposeful effort to tune in — *the circular route* — or through a spontaneous paranormal transmission — *the direct route.*)

This is also similar to the tuning-in and display process which takes place during a past life regression. The person remains connected physically and personally within the three dimensional context of his present life. However the screen on which consciousness is displayed has been tuned-in to accept the input from the fifth dimension. If we wish, we may call the display occurring on the screen through consciousness during a past life regression a psychogenetic memory which has been called forth from its warehouse or storage place.

The No-Field in the Quontic Field

The fifth dimensional quontic level doesn't have three dimensional type rules about time and space, energy and mass, light and speed, to regulate itself. We can't describe it adequately in three dimensional terms because its nature eludes three dimensional concepts and measurements. We know it exists because events and experiences occur continually in three dimensions even though empirical, scientific conceptualization cannot explain them. An explanation would require recourse to a dimension of invisible energies. However, using words and concepts can only be done in a three dimensional context, therefore, for fifth dimensional effects appearing in the third dimension a purely verbal description can never be absolutely true. Thus, we approximate a description by saying that time has no past, present or future, there is no intrinsic "arrow of time", space has no distance or direction, energy has no mass and mass has no energy, light has no speed, etc. Yet, like the electron, all have a tendency to exist, an action potential which can be activated by the proper preparatory and stimulating conditions, to manifest on the level of material reality and of consciousness.

The quotation from Newton's work at the beginning of this chapter intuitively foretold the transformation of wave into particle which led to quantum physics. It can also be viewed as a way of describing the transformation of energy from Harmonic into three dimensional consciousness, traversing the paranormal to the functional reality dimension. Newton's First Law of Motion and the Law of the Conservation of Energy have their origin in the fifth dimension where energy is neither created nor diminished, neither condensed nor expanded, but just is. The First Law states that "Every body continues in the state of rest or uniform motion in a straight line, except insofar as it is compelled by forces to change that state." (Gamow 1958[3]) That is to say, without forces such as friction, energy could continue an action in a straight line forever. More recently, it has been found that a form of energy called a soliton comes very close, but is not completely that ideal state. Solitons will be discussed in Part III.

Is it possible to have light that has no speed, or energy with no mass and no possibility of change? In other words, can there be a state of existence in which Conservation of Energy and the First Law of Motion operate in their pure states without restriction or change? Physics, operating under the constraints of rules limited to three dimensional interactions, poses itself an implicit conflict; it says it is not possible to draw those conclusions through empirical research, even though mechanically it postulates the conservation of energy, which in an ideal state never dissipates. Therefore, it conceives of an ideal state which is not measureable in itself which it says is responsible for states which are measureable. Conservation states that the forest turns to exhaust gases, ashes and heat when its wood is burned, changing its form but not its quantity. These may become invisible though they remain active in the universe, according to the Conservation of Energy law.

However, transformation of energy forms is not admitted by physics in the case of human psychic experience. The fact that non-measureable energies can have measureable effects in the three-dimensional universe is totally rejected by scientists only in dealing with paranormal phenomena. Later, in "The Purple Cow Dilemma", Chapter 8, it will be seen how scientists sometimes are compelled to accept but also arbitrarily reject concepts which have arisen in their own experimental paradigm because these concepts obstruct the conclusions that they have to produce in order to prove their theories. The concepts which they reject, as well as some they accept, do support the formulation of the paranormal model we are developing here. "The Quontic Field", on the quontic level, is what I have called the entire system that is specific to the fifth dimensional level of a no-field of functions, one that is non-measureable within its own domain but has very real effects in three dimensions.

Retrieval

Retrieval of information in quontic storage can be accomplished by tuning-in with the approriate resonance to the energy that is desired. The process is not easy because it has to have the correct resonance and has to pass through the fourth dimensional barrier in order to meet and draw the information, be it a healing energy, a spiritual quality or a past life memory from the unformed quontic to the formed, differentiated reality state.

Retrieval may be spontaneous or accompanied by a search process. Accessibility usually depends on gradual acceptance and skill in the attunement and retrieval process. Three-dimensional memories become stored in the everyday course of a lifetime; most are deeply buried in the unconscious and are not easily accessible to a person's here-and-now. The barrier of repression serves the purposes of leading an organized, non-chaotic daily life. Searching can be intentional, but intentionality, as we've seen, is not the only way that material may come back from the mundane unconscious. We are all familiar with trying to remember a person's name and, failing to do so, give up, only to have the name return to memory later. A once intentional search may be continued on a subconscious level even after conscious search has ceased. Searching to understand the environment as well as the self is part of the curiosity we see in animals and young children, as well as in adults. Searching appears to be a natural part of being alive, leading to the development and growth of very important aspects of the perceptual-cognitive functions of personality to determine what is and is not part of the self. An example of spontaneous searching for a recognizable, meaningful form is presented below, with a visually ambiguous pattern. (See Figure 13., *Penrose Tiles*,

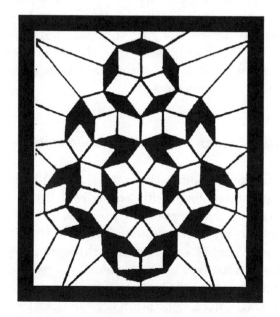

Figure 13.
Penrose Tiles,

obviously a cubic structure, restlessly changing its pattern as one attempts to extract meaning from it.

obviously a cubic structure, restlessly changing its pattern as one attempts to extract meaning from it.)

Consciousness loves to play with reality, to alter its forms and create new ones, to search for a new homeostasis. The degree to which it will do this depends on defense mechanisms and how rigidly they are in effect. In personality development, the play of consciousness has its full range of impact and effectiveness when barriers are not instituted against searching, beginning as early as childhood, within the spiritual and paranormal dimensions as part of the search for meaning.

The search function is an intrinsic part of the way human and animal experience in general serve the needs of the retrieval process. The means by which retrieval is accomplished physically is a complex biochemical and bioelectric psychoneurological process which has been woven through the tapestry of this book. We have been and will continue speculating about the scientific evidence available to describe the means by which the fifth dimensional aspect of the process occurs in order to describe it through its transformation via the quontic loop into a state recognizable in our mundane three dimensions.

Quantum Leap and Quontic Communications

What I'm describing in the concept of the quontic loop is something related to but different from the conventional quantum physical concept of the quantum leap. Very briefly, the "quantum leap" is a change in form that the electron may take between that of a presumably three-dimensional state called the particle and a non-dimensional yet measureable energy called a wave. Indeed, contemporary physics states there is not actually a separation between particle and wave, that they are both different aspects of the same thing. Somehow, they show up with different processes (see Chapter 7 on quantum physics in Part II for complete description of each), therefore are represented in terms of different information modes on detection equipment (see Chapter 8). Although they appear to be part of a single energy process, the shift from one to the other mode of functioning is sudden, precise and takes very different forms on detection equipment. However, it is relatively predictable and can be tracked by measuring devices and by means of quantum mechanical statistics.

Qualitatively, the descriptions of quantum mechanical processes and those of organic consciousness appear to have no relationship.

In the quontic system, each state (the three dimensional realistic and the fifth dimensional harmonic) may have its distinctive and different functions, capacities and processes, but apart from their differences there is also an intimate connectedness that we will perceive when we examine and describe their communication process. Through consciousness expansion skills, we have developed our access to their connectedness, learning to become a part of their intimate and special communication process. We don't have to take a statistical leap through quantum mechanics, we can judiciously enter the loop through consciousness.

I don't state that consciousness is a mental and psychic capability which exists as a part of the wave-particle shift, but that it seems to me that they are nevertheless intrinsic to one another, in different forms.

Von Neumann's assertion that the quantum leap is made by consciousness has been a tantalizing but rejected idea in physics. A "consciousness-created reality" school in physics (Herbert 1985 P.24[4] was started by von Neumann in 1932 with his book Die Grundlagen(von Neumann 1932[5]). Von Neumann, who is also responsible for developing the binary system used in modern computers, was a mathematician who demonstrated that electrons could not simply be ordinary three-dimensional particles and continue to function within the formulation of quantum theory. (We will see other formulations of this idea in Dirac's "sea of virtual electrons", in Bell's Theorem and again in Bohm's holographic theory.) If electrons were not ordinary particles neither could atoms which are made up of electrons be ordinary three-dimensional particles, so atoms could not be ordinary objects. Furthermore, if they were not ordinary objects they could not function under the ordinary laws of ordinary reality. This was not intended to deny the existence of ordinary reality but to state that it could not be directly inferred from quantum mechanics. Einstein was also unable to accept the notion that quantum mechanics was all there was to a description of reality, as we will see in the EPR Paradox.

Indeed, quantum physicists today accept the notion that atoms are not ordinary objects themselves, but are more like tendencies of energy to become something, and have energy sources outside of themselves. Nevertheless, since physics calls all of its descriptions absolutely realistic, there must be some accountability for the quantum leap, or what von Neumann called "the quantum wave collapse" into ordinary reality and he suggested that the most likely place that the change or the leap could occur is through the effect of consciousness.

At present there is no physical proof that consciousness has anything to do with the wave-particle problem, so it remains, at best for now, an undeveloped area, somewhere between the idea and its fact, in "potentia" in physics. However, other theories such as "Bell's Theorem", which will be taken up in Chapter 8, also has pointed physics, implicitly, in the direction of consciousness (Combs & Holland 1992[6]).

In sum, it appears that the quantum leap is an effect arising from the operation of the quontic loop.

The Fourth Dimension

I have suggested that the common boundary between the third and the fifth dimensions is the fourth dimension, which provides a barrier to the speed of light. In the quontic system the fourth dimension separates real and harmonic states of consciousness. Although channels of communication exist and are available between the 3D and the 5D states of consciousness, a boundary between them is not arbitrary but is predicated on the laws of the special theory of relativity. The fourth dimension incorporates time and space into a single dimension. Neither time nor space are invariable conditions, according to the special theory, and the main constant in the universe is the speed of light, 186,000 miles per second. In relativity, there is nothing beyond the fourth dimension. However quantum physics does not rest easily in this theoretical procrustean bed, it seems too short for the length and breadth of it. Relativity is also being stretched by the desire to unify all of physics into the Grand Unified Theory, needed to unify relativistic and quantum dynamics.

The boundary state given by the speed of light and the laws of relativity, effective as they are within their explanatory domain, also reflects limitations which creates a dilemma in quantum physics. When it is attempted to unify the four basic forces, (electromagnetism, gravity, and the strong and the weak forces), mathematical anomalies continually show up. Gravity cannot be unified, as yet, with the other three forces. Gravity is well integrated in relativity but gravity can still not be included in quantum mechanics because the attempt to unify them produces mathematical anomalies. Consequently, when mathematical infinities and negative energies show up in physics, it disrupts the quest for a grand unified theory of reality. Quantum physics has its own intrinsic "anomolies" as well, so a method has been devised that attempts to deal with these "anomolies" by "renormalizing" them because they would otherwise remain infinte, "impossible" quantities.

However, I will continue to point out how the "anomolies" are the basic stuff of a paradigm indicating the existence of a dimension which is non-linear in physics. The rejection of the anomalies frustrates the potential for a scientific formulation in both the GUT and in parapsychological studies. Their acceptance would not only unify physics and parapsychology, but could possibly lead to the Grand Unified Theory.

It is important to study the character of the boundary condition set up by relativity, particularly in its relationship to spiritual and parapsychological findings, and it is just as important to envisage the possibility that the relativistic boundary is not as impermeable as it appears. We will have more to say about this in Chapter 14, "Non-Linear Light Waves and Photonics". For now, it is important to continue exploring the meaning of quontic psychological dynamics.

Psychological Boundaries

In the quontic psychological model, the boundary condition in the fourth dimension disappears in the course of unconscious, spontaneously natural and unprogrammed processes resulting in observations of harmonic consciousness which take place at the detection screen of human consciousness. We will consider briefly how this occurs when we discuss how responses to the electromagnetic waves of the external environment impinge on the electromagnetic waves of the internal environment in a state of resonance.

Energy arrives at the detection screen (neurophysiologically the brain, body, feeling, mind network; psychologically consciousness) of the person from two sources of information. One source is its psychoneurophysiological system which gives rise to reality consciousness and the other source is the fifth dimension and the quontic warehouse which give rise to harmonic consciousness. The two systems of information, the harmonic and the realistic, contribute energy to nervous system impulses which then constitute a patterned network of internally and externally derived associations which become displayed within consciousness. The boundary between harmonic and reality consciousness and between external and internal communication processes can be bridged intentionally by developing skills that open and maintain resonance in channels of access to harmonic consciousness.

Research has shown that only a small portion of the totality of psychological stimuli surrounding us is detected consciously, the rest is either absorbed unconsciously or not allowed admission. Stimuli from either harmonic or reality consciousness can be rejected as a psychological foreign body in the same way the immune system is biologically programmed to reject invasion from foreign cells. However, both mind and body can make serious errors in determining what is or is not a foreign body. Developmental personality processes, through the use of the ego and reality consciousness, help determine what the person will or will not regard as a foreign body. However, psychologically as well as physically, sometimes the body's own necessary, vital parts and functions are considered "foreign", rejected, and destroyed or disabled. Physiologically autoimmune diseases and psychologically self-destructive behavior which harm the mind and body are outcomes of rejecting the self as an alien body or rejecting the body as alien to the self. There has been some investigation of a psychological aspect to the autoimmune system which acts destructively against the psychological as well as the physical organism, during work done in cancer and some in AIDS. Further psychophysiological research is needed in this area.

Differentiation and discrimination by a person between "bodies" that are truly invasive and harmful and those that are positive or benign is consonant with maximal physical and emotional awareness. Positive and negative stimuli can then be dealt with consciously, accurately identified as beneficial or harmful, and responses can be directed in a purposeful way instead of with lack of control due to lack of or misdirected conscious awareness.

In the quontic system, effective conscious psychophsiological awareness comes about through contact with the Organic Self. Awareness of body-mind connections is inherent in the functioning of a healthy Organic Self. Consciousness is open to it when it is not blocked off by defense mechanisms. The Organic Self is a part of the body that is capable of differentiating and communicating its true state, that is, whether the person is being aggressed by toxic stimuli or is subjected to nourishing input. Many psychological problems are the outcome of the inability to differentiate stimuli beginning at the organic level.

The strongest defense against toxic stimuli and against misidentifying such stimuli occurs when information processed by the Organic Self of the person is open to stimuli from the various physiological parts of the body. Internal facilitation of neurophysiological communication processes will send information from the Organic Self to Reality Consciousness where conscious awareness will be able to absorb, process, and make appropriate decisions about the information. This information processing can be enhanced by access to energy from the harmonic dimension.

In the healing process, fifth dimensional Harmonic Consciousness serves to provide an additional interface with three dimensional Reality Consciousness via the quontic loop. The bridge between harmonic and reality consciousness is vital to a wholistic concept of health. It is not a matter of which consciousness is better, a conflict promoted by people on each side of it, because ultimately integrating and bridging both levels of consciousness is necessary for total well-being.

Once admitted as a friendly, acceptable stimulus (even when reception in the physical body is totally unconscious), what the person receives from harmonic consciousness can finally become further organized as memories in the internal brain-mind environment. When the unconscious itself is receptive to stimuli from harmonic consciousness, the received stimuli can be stored as unconscious memories including those it has differentiated as toxic or non-toxic stimuli. The memories may be projected into consciousness in dreams or recalled intentionally as part of the survival and homeostatic drive and perhaps can appear at other times when the guardianship of defensive mechanisms is lowered.

Memories with their connections at both ends of the quontic loop are essential to homeostasis. Memories become information, and depending on the kind of memory involved, can lead to the kind of data bank we call knowledge. Memories are personal and affect emotions and self-concept, normally with positive results when they are directed by homeostasis toward centeredness. On the other hand, if developmental memories are overwhelmingly feared and repressed by defense mechanisms, the psychophysical and the fifth-dimensional quontic field of the body-mind may lose their capacity for synchronization and therefore the body-mind's ability to perform with effective homeostatic interactions becomes stressed, and sometimes altogether wiped out. Psychological and/or physical disease is the outcome.

On the three-dimensional psychophysiological level of body-mind, homeostasis is stressed when the information available in memories through feedback conflicts with the feelings and self-image, or self-concept, which a person wants to maintain and project to others. Defense mechanisms prevent integration of memories and self-image within the psychophysical body-mind, i.e. consciousness. If defense mechanisms overwhelm the organic self, it will not be able to communicate its information to the next level and the homeostatic mechanism will not be able to perform its function. Homeostasis will not be able to move the person from a stressed position to an equilibrious one. The body-mind, with its blocked feelings and distorted self-concept under a consistently stressed condition enters into a dysfunctional state of neurosis and/or physical illness. It's on red-alert when, despite the state of warning that the system is off-balance, the psychophysiological collaboration natural to the immune system's protective devices can't return it to equilibrium on their own. Professional help is then vitally needed.

To sum it up, one part of homeostasis and of consciousness has a transpersonal form of operation in the universe, and is therefore meta-physical; the other part has a personalized form and is psychophysical. Nevertheless, they interact. The degree of interaction depends on the tuning-in process. In the Yogic system of thought two intertwining snakes represent the interaction between the psychophysical and the metaphysical aspects of consciousness. They are depicted running from the first chakra in the pelvis to the seventh chakra in the crown of the head, implicating the entire body as the vessel for consciousness. The tuning-in is done through meditation in Yoga. The medical profession has taken the intertwined snakes, the caduceous, for its symbol but has ignored the heart of it, the meaning of consciousness collaborating with the body. However, both parts, psychophysical and meta-physical bodies, are necessarily interactive and must be integrated in order to maximize a person's health.

In its maximized healthy state, the total context of the conscious mind is made up of all psychophysical and metaphysical parts. People who fragment the physical from the psychological and metaphysical parts functionally talk of the physical and medical cause of an illness as if that rules out any psychological or spiritual component. There is even the attempt to turn mind into a purely physiologically explained phenomenon.

What we mean when we talk about total or unifunctional consciousness is that we have developed awareness which arose out of information we received from the total informational feedback system from both its harmonic and its reality sources which are in a state of resonance within our bodies. Our bodies are the channels through which we receive information relevant to itself as a part of our psychological selves as well as information about the state of other people, or even about the universe. What is initially available varies among people and can be readily increased through consistent experiences and training which open mind, body, feelings and self-concept to further information from both reality and harmonic consciousness.

Whether Quontic Psychology makes sense is not a scientific matter, or concern, at present. It is sufficient for it to serve the purpose of making people more comfortable and accepting of spiritual and parapsychological experience that may have confused or frightened them. If the person exploring these questions finds it easier to live within a self-concept that includes an expanded-reality orientation, and is able to integrate the "irrational" into the consciousness of a sane human being, then Quontic Psychology has fulfilled its goal.

Glossary of Terms Used in Quontic Psychology

QUONTIC PSYCHOLOGY

A comprehensive explanation of paranormal, scientific, psychological and spiritual experience integrating concepts in Psychology, Physics, Neurophysiology and Metaphysics, as well as other sciences into the Field of Complex Unity Studies, thereby becoming a model for integrating concepts from a great variety of studies to better understand humankind's place and potential in relation to himself and the universe.

1. Three-Dimensional Field Concepts

ORGANIC SELF

Physiological impulses, sensations and drives, a body-oriented self which attempts to input information into the Real Self for use in consciousness. A vital level of organismic functioning - it dominates in childhood and is sublimated in maturity. If repeatedly ignored and repressed it's message of dysfunctional homeostasis comes through as physical or mental illness.

REAL SELF

Nourished by the Organic Self, its physiological impulses are organized on a somewhat higher level of complexity. Transformed into feelings and emotions and organized into a self-concept with the help or hindrance of the Ego. It is often repressed along with the Organic Self. It nevertheless has a subtlety in its basic energy that makes demands for attention through slips, dreams, illnesses and accidents when its communications passed on from the Organic Self are not overtly accepted by the Ego.

EGO

The arbitrator between the demands of the Real Self and the Idealized Self, regulated on the one hand by Defense Mechanisms working on behalf of the Idealized Self and

Homeostatic Mechanisms working on behalf of the Real Self. Its position is therefore often one of conflict, confusion, and fear about not fulfilling the demands of each and/or fulfilling demands of one at the expense of the other. All of that and trying to deal with outer reality too makes the Ego vulnerable to breakdowns.

IDEALIZED SELF

The product of shoulds, should-nots, frustrations and demands of parents and peers during developmental years, created with the assistance of the superego. When a child tries to satisfy social goals and strivings, an idealized image is often constructed on a foundation of defense mechanisms and not organic feelings, thus often is self-deluded into believing it's allied with reality and the real self simultaneously. It is therefore unfortunately also able to create blindness about unreal, psychopathic and neurotic behavior, using defense mechanisms.

It may nevertheless contain suppressed ideals that are constructive and valuable motivating positive social actions and psychotherapeutic intervention for help in fulfilling itself.

DEFENSE MECHANISMS

Self-protective devices with complex dynamics which may encapsulate the real self, block sensations and the expression of emotions, distort perceptual and cognitive functions, in the service simultaneously of an idealized self and a dysfunctional ego. Possibly needed at one time for survival during developmental years, it may continue in full capacity when no longer relevant to situations, instigating inappropriate, repetitious, neurotic behavior during adulthood. The cement of defense mechanisms is unconscious, developmentally induced, fear and anger which also provide an incentive to cling to old perceptions and behavior. Wards off attempts to change old, "tried and true" ways for new perceptions that would threaten its hegemony, therefore a major opponent of psychotherapy and other change processes.

REALITY CONSCIOUSNESS

An ally and source of information for the ego which may or may not be open to new resources for information. Functioning on the three-dimensional side of consciousness, it may or may not be open to channels through feedback loops to Harmonic Consciousness, depending on strength and focus of defense mechanisms. When healthy, is amenable to adjustments in reality perceptions due to reception of information through life experiences, scientific method, adjustments and improvements in alignment of memories and current personal experience, from reality testing and intuition, and from the Harmonic Self.

CURRENT LIFE MEMORIES

Memories of all current life events returning to childhood, infancy, birth and the womb, recallable both intentionally and spontaneously under appropriate conditions. Except for resistance found after Defense Mechanisms are formed, these are instrumental in influencing all the above components in the development of personality. Essential for maintainance of homeostasis and survival.

3D SPACE-TIME

The conventional world of Newtonian functioning which determines socially accepted reality. A major influence on reality consciousness, but not the only one.

FOURTH DIMENSION

The unification of space and time in relativity theory; a boundary condition between the third and fifth dimensions defined by the speed of light in quontic psychological theory. In the latter, it can be transcended by appropriate physical and/or psychological transformations.

HOMEOSTASIS

A balancing of energies within a given range on the 3D level of all of the forces acting on a person promoting survival, growth and change. Capable of evolving along with evolutionary forces by using feedback and memory systems whose products arise out of fundamental experiences in survival.

HOMEOSTATIC PRINCIPLE

A fundamental regulatory principle found in every aspect of existence from the cosmic to the microcosmic, balancing forces and energies within a certain range enabling organic as well as inorganic systems to maintain their capacity to function. It operates, along with feedback and mnemonic sensitivities between third and fifth dimensions in the quontic loop.

FEEDBACK

A psychophysiological system, employing electromagnetic, biochemical, psychobioneurological processes to communicate information to various parts of the organism, necessary for homeostasis and survival.

2. Quantic Field — Fifth Dimension Concepts

QUONTIC MEMORIES

When accessed through transformational dynamics, facilitates paranormal experiences such as the return to prior existing lifetimes, bypassing 4th dimensional, speed of light boundary conditions to retrieve pastlife information for use in the contemporary timeframe of the regressor. Can afford knowledge of the universe on a broader than simply human level, accessible through the Quontic Loop.

QUONTIC FIELD

A non-physically definable area of the universe in which quontic relationships occur, viz: no temporal or spacial differentiations into past, present and future time or near and far; acausal, non-linear, supraluminal communications are characteristic. May also be regarded as the implicate domain in Bohm's holographic concept and the domain of

Universal Oneness of Eastern mysticism. However, it is derived equally importantly in this formulation from concepts in physics, neuropsychology and other sciences which have not yet heretofore been integrated into an adequate wholistic theory. Separated by the fourth dimension from conventional 3D activities.

QUONTIC LOOP

Facilitates communications as an energy channel between the third and fifth dimensions. Serves as a feedback loop for information between the two dimensions by permitting energy transformations to occur in energetic contexts which ordinarily separate the two dimensions.

QUONTICLE

Any entity, no matter how small or large, that can exhibit both wave and particle aspects as in quantum physics. As such, it serves as the vehicle for transporting energy in the quontic loop between 3D and 5D.

QUON

The unformed energy itself carried by the quonticle before it becomes either wave or particle in its ultimately measureable form.

PARENCHYMA

The organic aspect of 5D, a self-generating, self perpetuating source of organic life energy pervading everything. It is accessible through transformations of energy to communicate information, but cannot be described as being in, for, or about, anything. It just is and the rest follows. Strongly connected, perhaps the energetic source for, a universal homeostatic energy that keeps the universe in a balanced state despite variations due to movements and changes. Can manifest itself as aspects of Harmonic Self and Consciousness in human functioning.

HARMONIC SELF

The highest developmental level of spiritual orientation possible for Harmonic Consciousness. Its function and mode of operation when accessed is to establish the connection to a state of homeostasis within and surrounding an energy field, human or otherwise. When translated into three dimensional communications, its experiential energy is commonly described as "universal peace", "universal love", "spiritual love", etc.

The awareness level for the harmonic self is aptly described as a source of inner guidance and inner wisdom, peaceful and loving feelings and well-being. The experience occurs through "tuning in" to something larger than daily consciousness and by developing awareness that will transcend the barrier to self-realization. The psychophysiological level of consciousness is the receiver and display screen for communications from the harmonic self via the quontic loop. When such communications are fully effective, they can be transmitted to reality consciousness and to the organic self thus becoming an ongoing part of desirable and healthy personality changes.

This is the kind of experience which defies conventional scientifically determinable validation and despite that is validated experientially every day by millions of people within and outside of traditional religion and spiritual organizations. If science had a paradigm that accepted human experience it would end the issue.

Consciousness Squared on Skyros

After a while you learn the subtle difference
Between holding a hand and chaining a soul
And you learn that love doesn't mean leaning
And company doesn't mean security,
And you begin to learn that kisses aren't contracts
And presents aren't promises,
And you begin to accept your defeats
With your head up and your eyes open,
With the grace of a (man or) woman,
Not the grief of a child
And learn to build all your roads
On today because tomorrow's ground
is too uncertain for plans, and futures have
A way of falling down in mid-flight.
After awhile you learn that even sunshine
Burns if you get too much.
So you plant your own garden and decorate
Your own soul, instead of waiting
For someone to bring you flowers,
And you learn that you really can endure...
That you really are strong
And you really do have worth.
And you learn and learn...
With every goodbye you learn.

— Anonymous

Reality Testing in Psychotherapy

My search for a larger, paranormal reality is a process which engages a good part of my therapy work as well as my participation in the society surrounding me. This is a search that leads of necessity to unconventional ideas about reality. Unconventional ideas are native to alternative psychotherapy processes such as those utilized within Organic Process Therapy. An acknowledged problem with alternative therapies is whether they have criteria to demonstrate whether they are realistically effective in assisting clients.

The quontic psychological paradigm presented in the last chapter is an attempt make rational something that is intrinsically irrational. The effort is necessary however because there are applications in the healing process as well as in daily life that are important for healthy human functioning.

Conventional ideas about health are based on science which has its problems in communicating with the irrational side of the thought process. However, that is what is necessary for the maintainance of homeostasis. As we've already seen in the psychobioneurological ideas that have been investigated by science, conscious thought is only the tip of the iceberg of what constitutes the construction of consciousness. Like von Neumann's ideas about the electron, without the irrational aspect of it you would not have the part that you can see and deal with consciously—without the wave the electron would not exist in the real world.

Alternative healing depends to a far greater extent than other kinds of treatment on accessibility to the unifunctional bodymind for its success. To use it therefore takes an openness to the irrational. The doublebind here is that openness to the irrational creates anxiety in a normally functioning individual; however, it can be dealt with as another aspect of the process. There are claims to reality that have to be respected and met in the course of expanding and opening to other aspects of it. Otherwise, homeostasis can get thrown too far off balance too quickly for it to cope with changes.

In other words, therapy has to be realistic in the sense that it matches the needs of the particular client if it is to help him to shift his self-concept and his mode of functioning into a more serviceable homeostasis. The question is, what criteria do we have to evaluate the capacity to deal with reality on the part of either the therapy process or the client in an alternative process? These are some of the concerns that will be taken up in the presentation of several case histories in this chapter. An overall concern is to recognize when a paranormal experience during a session is indeed a fundamental part of it, and when it is not and may serve a defensive or neurotic purpose. The following are criteria which seem appropriate.

The paranormal aspect can be considered reliable if the person's overall functioning is also accompanied by:

1. A strong enough grounding in conventional reality to manifest a high degree of awareness and concern for interpersonal relationships and the multiple variety of possibilities inherent in them. Joining with others in groups or friendships to share experiences, gain and offer support, establish values, for example.

2. A fundamental ability to understand and cope with problems successfully enough during therapy to lead to personal growth. The enjoyment of personal growth without, or minimal, guilt or self-punishment.

3. The manifestation of a thoughtful curiosity and sense of challenge about the paranormal and spiritual dimensions. The self-concept can absorb the necessary changes in self-image that accompany new values.

4. When a person's reality testing is an intrinsic mode of functioning he can enjoy the challenges, discoveries and adventures that accompany him on the path of paranormal

and spiritual exploration without losing contact with everyday reality. The ego shows enough flexibility to relish the
search while carefully evaluating the reality considerations.

This is very different from the reality of a person who is
severely neurotic in which there is a flimsy contact with
reality to begin with and a severe, potentially traumatic
break is already present in the unconscious which motivates
distortions in daily behavior and in the perception of others'
behavior. It's true that such persons may or may not also
have strong contact with fifth dimensional energies but there
are important distinctions to be made which will be brought
out in this chapter through case histories.

Perhaps this next point has to be made more strongly. It's
that reality testing does not rest solely within the province
of the physical sciences. The methods of reality testing used
by the physical sciences do not apply, or applies only in a
limited way to the social sciences, and least of all to psychotherapy in particular. Reality testing for psychotherapy is
a province governed by experienced changes in the life of the
person who is in therapy. When I receive verbal or written
reports of behavioral changes that have dramatically im-
proved a client's life, changed that person's awareness and
expanded his success in interpersonal relationships, I am
certain of the proven reality value of the hypotheses with
which I treat them. However, the laboratory in such a case
is organic, dynamic and vital and depends on changes that
can happen only once rather than being mechanistic, statistical and robotically repeatable.

Nevertheless, the success of psychotherapy, especially
when using transpersonal methods, opens the door to new
questions regarding the fundamental basis for the success.
In fact it was such questioning that made a book such as this
necessary. Nor can I always say that I have secure answers
that enable me to understand why the positive changes
occurred in every case. Following are two cases which are
examples of situations in which I am certain of the reality

value of the solutions since the behavior involved rapidly changed for the better but I remained open to a better hypothesis about the immediate causes of change. In general, they fit into the model of quontic psychology and the drawing upon energies which run the gamut of the quontic loop, but neither were solutions that arose from past life or my other familiar styles of conducting Organic Process Therapy. Here I present them with questions in mind about the cause of change.

Organic Process at the Skyros Centre

In Aug. 1991 I went for the sixth non-consecutive year to work for two weeks at the Skyros Center on the island of Skyros, Greece. It is exciting to work there because of the calibre of clients who come from all over Europe and because of their generally extremely high motivation to cut through to the source of their problems. It makes my work, which is done in small groups of eight to fifteen persons usually, more intense, sometimes more risky, and much more gratifying than working at places where clients are too anxious about getting upset to penetrate more than superficial levels of defenses. Good, durable therapy depends on an effective collaboration between client and therapist. The desire for a miracle-like cure itself is testimony to an encapsulated personality that would make in-depth self-exploration and durable change difficult to reach.

There was, in fact, during the second of these two weeks a person who had a superficially intact persona with an apparently psychotic underlay. The potential for psychosis began to reflect itself in severe distortions of the meaning of the therapy process with accusations showing she felt her survival was endangered. Later she spoke without feeling about a dream in which she identified herself as a person who had been killed. It became clear that developmental life threatening circumstances had been triggered and transferred themselves as an encapsulated reality into the present.

(Other group members had been dealing with life and death issues, as will be seen in the following case histories.) Under these circumstances, she could not be treated in the context of the group process. She wanted "spiritual healing" she said but wouldn't commit herself as a participant to the healing process, which requires the assumption of personal responsibilty and not supra-human miracles. Her presence, in fact, became so stressed that she interfered with the treatment of the other group members, thinking they were being harmed. Finally, after some difficulty, I enabled her to leave the group process without uprooting her psychosis, leaving her feeling intact and able to function. She even said later that it was a valuable experience.

The events described above occurred next to the last days of my work with a particular group. It furthered the need to discriminate between people whose psychoses don't show ordinarily through their defenses, but in fact whose "spiritual work" is a defense against potential psychosis, compared to those who have the ego strength to genuinely want to let their deeply buried internal problems come into the light of day to facilitate healing. The second type of person may look sicker on the surface due to the overt expression of pain or anger but can also be the healthier person in strength of access and ability to cope with emotions needed for their own healing process. With accessibility to emotional conflicts there is then possible a positive outcome for the resolution of internal-external conflicts and the restoration of a better level of homeostasis in daily functioning.

On the last day, there was one example of a therapy case that I worked with that provided a satisfying example of the distinction between neurotic and healthy alternative processes in which spiritual energy could be brought to bear upon problems in daily functioning. As indicated earlier, this group of people were functioning at better than average levels in general, even though they also had experienced traumatic unfinished business in their personal lives. We had, during my week in this group, already experienced a person's extraordinary recollection and reliving of a suicide attempt and had accessed from unconscious memory two spontaneous birth primals of very different kinds, both of which were triggered by the reexperiencing of the attempted suicide. In fact they occurred in quick succession creating an unusually difficult therapy situation.

In each session, although the events of the trauma are recounted as experienced and relived by one group member, there is a real sense of group sharing of responsibility for the processing and outcome after sharing traumatic events. In this way, life and death had become reality issues for the members of this group. Their mutually supportive level of awareness helped in coping very successfully with the issues that were brought up. Several were able to function as therapeutic assistants while their counterparts were reexperiencing the suicide attempt and birth primals. The persons who received the direct help reported feeling relaxed, cared about, more loving, more able to be with others after discharging such trauma and receiving caring themselves from the other group members.

Lisa's Son

On the last day, another person who had not worked as yet, said that there was a death that she had never fully dealt with. We'll call her Lisa. It was the accidental drowning of her son. Her life, she felt, was in abeyance since his death. Lisa had been successful as a mental health practioner, had belonged to groups, had warm relationships, but had given up internally, lost energy and had almost totally discontinued her practice in a state of depression. When asked for details about her son's death, she said he was in his late teens, was a scuba diver and it happened while they were on a holiday. She was present at the site when he drowned. As she recounted the details, presenting an image of herself standing on a pier waiting for the boat to return coming back without him, her eyes filled with tears saying she felt she had never grieved for him. Lisa was tall and stately and was a loving mother figure for the other group members, and everyone rallied to her support. I saw her as a person with a great deal of spiritual connection with her son and she had indeed recounted several episodes in which ESP seemed to have been a mode of communication between them.

To her surprise, I told her I thought she needed to separate herself from him, that she had not yet done so. Perhaps he had not separated from her either since people dying traumatic deaths involuntarily don't seem to realize they are dead and have to leave the earth plane for another level of existence, I said. Her eyes widened fearfully and she wanted to know if it was the only way she could get relief from her grief and I told her it was the best way that I knew. She agreed to try.

I felt that she didn't need a lot of breathing relaxation and imaging exercises, which I frequently use, and asked her whether she could feel her son's presence. After a few moments she said she could and indeed I visualized a young man in shorts and T-shirt saying "Hi, Mum". At any rate, his presence seemed palpable. However, she visualized him not as a solid person, not describing him dressed as I had seen him, but as made up of a kind of "stardust" sparkling material. He was not surrounded by objects and was transparent, but very real to her nevertheless. After a few moments, with my prompting, she began talking to him, weeping profusely, telling him how much she loved him, how terrible she felt about his death and that she missed him very much. After this went on for some time, I prompted her again about saying goodbye, upon which she said to him that she needed to say goodbye to him. With one hand poised in the air, she reported that she saw a long (umbilical?) cord connecting herself to her son and that she would have to cut it before he could leave. Her weeping intensified as she moved her hand in a gesture of cutting the cord. The group participants were totally empathic, some were weeping, others were comforting her or each other. Thereafter she grew silent as if she were watching him leaving the earth plane. When she looked up she wanted to know if he would be happy and I assured her he would be.

During the discussion, following the general sharing of personal feelings within the group process, Lisa said she felt good about the experience and felt she would, on returning home, become freer to do what she wanted to do for herself in her own life. She said she had known there was somethng important for her to do in the group, but didn't know what it was until this morning. She was grateful I was able to help her. I subsequently heard from her and from other group members to the effect that she had resumed her life in full.

The question of neurotic behavior is not even at issue here, in my opinion. This woman's concern and the group's concern for her was totally in a realistic context of need awareness and bonding in interpersonal relationships. Her ability to access fifth dimensional energies was something she brought with her into the group and the safety provided by knowing I accepted and worked with such energies helped her to present it for therapeutic intervention. The loss of her son probably made her a more loving person in the group and her group acceptance probably gave her the additional security she needed to trigger her recall and release her emotions about her son's death.

The reality question might be asked whether he was really present in spirit. I have no proof but I think he was. In fact, the description she gave of his body reminded me of the kind of spirit energy or etheric body that was described by another client with whom I worked while I was in Brazil.

On the side of the skeptics is the fact that Lisa's attachment to her son was very powerful and emotionally she had not let go. The dialogue with him could be explained as a familiar Gestalt exercise in which she simply imagined her son's presence, the umbilical cord was a perfect symbol for the exercise, and cutting it accomplished its goal of enabling her to release herself from her possessiveness and from the grief about his death - all symbolically. It was good therapy and not contact with a spirit being.

That this person formed good social contact, was herself
well grounded in reality, had real empathic relationships
with others and was dealing with episodic, not chronic neurotic behavior was further data countering the assumption
that the spiritual aspect was a fantasy projection of a chronic
neurotic person who lacked contact with reality. The outcome, the resumption of her life following the therapy process
speaks for itself in favor of the alternative aspect.

Psychic Placebo or Healing?:
The Case of "The Wobbly"

At first, I didn't know whether to include "The Wobbly"
because I didn't know what to make of it, but at a farewell
dinner from Skyros island some of the participants were
joking about the strange manner in which the healing of one
participant came about, and then I realized that the fact that
I can't explain it is no reason not to include it. The session
took place on the second day of the second week at Skyros,
in the same group as the case recounted above.

This participant complained of a pain in her stomach that
had bothered her for many months which got better and
worse but never completely went away. It limited her eating,
she couldn't tolerate foods that were "wobbly" (foods that
weren't hard). It interfered with her bowel movements. At
present it had become very painful and now she could hardly
eat anything at all. It was centered in her stomach. When
I asked her to describe it she said it was something that
wobbled around inside her and she couldn't grasp it. It was
an unappetizing yellow or greenish color, like bile. She
physically tried to touch it but reported that it moved around
inside her whenever she seemed to approach it so that it
always eluded her grasp.

When I asked her to have a dialogue with it she didn't,
reverting back to describing it and telling her experience of
it. When I requested associations, hoping for a memory about

a painful experience during childhood she could come up with nothing. Nevertheless, her pain was very real, her desire to work it out was genuine, and her attempt to grasp it psychologically and physically were totally frustrated. It was a very difficult situation because all the usual methods that I employ in my attempts to help my clients were to no avail. It was just as evasive to me as it was to her.

Without thinking too much about it, I said I would help her look for it and began feeling around her midsection, putting some slight pressure at various points. When I came to a point on her left side she began to scream in pain and I gloated "I found it, here it is!" I continued to put pressure at that point while she groaned in pain, and then I said that I would take it out of her and made movements as if pulling something out of her side and throwing it away. After three or four minutes of this kind of movement I returned to the reactive pressure point and pressed again. The pain was much reduced though not altogether gone, she said. I repeated the movements and when I went back to it again it was almost gone.

I decided to let it go at that but offered her a group healing which she accepted. In this exercise each member of the group sits around a person who is stretched out on the floor, says a prayer for the subject's well-being and prays for recovery from whatever is ailing them while moving their hands over the subject without touching. Each member of the group took a turn doing this. This is similar to the practice of laying on of hands which I also appreciated through my experiences with psychic surgery.

For the rest of the week until the end of the session this participant remained well. She said that the pain left her completely the following day. Her appetite returned, she could once again eat foods that had made her feel sick before and her bowel movements became normal again. Color had returned to her face. Since she was normally an attractive, athletic woman her appearance returned to her pre-illness attractiveness and vigor. After that she was very firm in supporting others in going through their own difficulties in the group.

She asked for an explanation of what I did and I couldn't tell her for sure. It was not Gestalt therapy or Psychodrama or recall through psychophysiological regression, and it certainly wasn't past life therapy, any of which could have become useful in her state normally, but weren't. That left either the placebo effect of attributing magical powers to me which enabled her to believe she was being cured of her ailment or psychic healing in which I was able to call forth healing powers in myself and subsequently enabled the group to use their powers as well to cure her pain. In either case, this woman was transformed from a state of unhappy complaints to lively and valuable participation for the rest of her stay. I prefer to believe that a calling forth of psychic energies helped her, as well as the other participants.

Again, this was another woman functioning well, holding down a responsible position in her career, who had no history of hysterical diagnostic complaints, but who suffered this one episodic painful event which responded, I believe, to purely psychic healing. Further than that, I can't demonstrate a proof of how she was cured but I favor an explanation that draws upon the powers of the connections between the physical body with its very specific mode of functioning and the resources available in the psychic domain. The body and the feelings were operating in concert to inform the person that homeostasis was badly off center.

Her body's own drive for restoration of homeostatic balance was self-evident. What threw her balance off into the dysfunctional state that developed was not discovered. Nevertheless, a connection to the Organic Self was communicated and within this context it is possible to access the connection to fifth dimensional healing sources. Her pain had established a resonance within herself that made necessary the access she gained to higher level functions for healing. Later chapters will further expand upon and clarify what terms such as these mean.

Considering the intensive scientific studies still to come, the material that has been presented up until now has been easy. The following few chapters are an attempt to review some fundamental ideas in quantum physics and relativity theory from the point of view of how they fit in with Quontic Psychology. These subjects are never facile in their translation from physics to ordinary daily English. Therefore, for our purposes, I have sought some sort of compromise between scientific and everyday language structure - not diluting the scientific information, yet attempting to condense and clarify as well as could be expected.

It has been done before so why do it again? Quantum physics lends itself to metaphysical concepts, as has been the reflection of a number of excellent books on the subject. It will be valuable if the reader has already perused some of these books because prior grounding will make what follows more readable. (Capra 1975, Talbot 1981, Davies, 1982, and others - see references.)

The early portion of Part 2, the chapter on quantum physics, introduces some fundamentals which are basically well known and may seen repetitious, but this groundwork is needed for the more critical evaluation of physics in "The Purple Cow" chapter. If it seems too heavy, read for the overall picture that you can get out of it. The scientific details, for our purposes, are not that crucial. Rereading at your leisure will help to clarify the ideas considerably. With that apologia to all out of the way, let's get on with it.

Part II

Quantum Physics:
The Holes
Within
The Whole

Quantum Physical Reality

"In the face of the lack of direct mathematical demonstration, one must be careful and thorough to make sure of the point, and one should make a perpetual attempt to demonstrate as much of the formula as possible. Nevertheless, a very great deal more truth can become known than can be proven."

— Richard Feynman,
Nobel Prize in Physics,
acceptance address, 1965.

The Expansion of Science

Something intriguing about quantum physics compels physics writers exploring the fringe of connections between scientific and paranormal phenomena to link quantum physics and meta-physics. My first excitement due to seeing something familiar about the relationship occurred listening to a lecture by Fritjof Capra in New York in the early 1970's, and I soon realized this was a more sophisticated variation on the conversational themes that a physicist friend, Jean Louis Cattaui and I had been having in the 1960's before his death.

Quantum theory really makes it necessary to formulate basically new ideas about the nature of reality. These new ideas challenge a Newtonian reality which is always predictable and knowable, given adequate data for experimental procedures. Instead it opens the door to ideas which question the role of the experimenter in determining his data and therefore his view of reality, and makes uncertain the amount of data reality is willing to relinquish at any one moment.

Additionally, there is a great deal of information arriving from inadequately knowable sources, such as "virtual photons", "solitons", "zero point energy", "non-linear spacetime", "faster-than-light communications" and so on, some of which are in limbo because they cannot be integrated into even the unconventional ideas of quantum physics. For the most part, these latter "impossible conclusions", as we shall call them, are not yet proven facts in scientific reality though some are statistically verifiable forms of information. However, from the quontic psychological standpoint they are intriguing developments arising out of proven theories which could ultimately extend those theories beyond the confines of their experimentally proven data. For instance, non-linear spacetime allows time to go backward. Physicists like Stephan Hawking conjecture about the possibility of this happening if you take quantum theory to its limits. Communications that transcend lightspeed's limits are ruled out for atoms in relativity theory in three and four dimensional space but not for atoms in another, fifth or higher dimension of existence in non-linear quantum speculation. If true, this would have very important significance for the reality of fifth-dimensional, paranormal phenomena in general and for past life regression in particular.

In this chapter we will examine what contemporary quantum physics says by means of large brushstrokes to see how it interprets reality in ways that are acceptable to most physicists as well as those ideas in it that give it a non-ordinary, "beyond the quantum" potential. We will then look at how reality begins to take a shape that can be interpreted as meta-physical yet keep its data, if we move the kaleidoscope of our perceptual apparatus an additional small turn to the right - or to the left if you will think of it politically - to include its rejected data into expanded concepts.

Our purpose is to find out more about ideas that share a common ground between science, consciousness and metaphysics. This would enable us to develop a firmer foundation for Quontic Psychology and ultimately enable us to relate to paranormal experience as another aspect of both scientific and everyday life.

We have already been able to introduce ideas which have led us to see that the concept of homeostasis provides a common ground for the physical and psychological aspect of human and other organic forms of functioning. Non-organic and mechanical systems in general also can be described as being dependent on homeostatic devices for their successful ongoing operation.

Does physics, and quantum physics in particular, have anything to offer in this vein of a commonality with the homeostasis found in other studies in the sciences? There are a number of things that suggest it, but perhaps the strongest is a notion that has become very central in physics, the notion of symmetry, or taking its longer name, the symmetry group of nature. This will be expanded some in this chapter, and further still in Chapter 12, "Symmetry and It's Breaking".

Underlying the mathematical predictions of all quantum physics is the factor of uncertainty. In itself, prediction from uncertainty sounds like an inherent contradiction, but the need to resolve issues arising from such yin-yang kinds of polarities that look like opposites is what quantum physics has been evolving from. It's as if you can give uncertainty a structure that provides you with the predictability that gives you the experience of the everyday world as it is. From uncertainty comes predictability. Recently, chaos theory has come up with the same kind of observations and its own kind of explanatory mathematics to describe how chaos is the forerunner of highly organized patterns and processes. It seems that chaos itself has an underlying structure which propels it toward the organization of matter into the formal processes that we observe and live with everyday. That theme is repeated in many different ways in physics, as reliably as human behavior reproduces Freud's notion of the repetition compulsion.

With all this new information about chaos and uncertainty, it seems simultaneously even more and less amazing that the highly organized world of Newtonian Physics could have ever been extracted from nature. However, conventional reality becomes more explicable when we perceive homeostasis as the underlying energy that drives the mundane universe. Homeostasis allows for the occurrence of apparently unpredictable, chaotic phenomena - perhaps the Big Bang was such an "unpredictable" phenomenon; and at the same time it is underlyingly acting to change and reorganize the outward effects of events in the course of their interactions. It is this factor of an underlying organizing function, the symmetry described by Weinberg, which we will find equivalent to the homeostatic principle. Then, with a turn of the kaleidoscope we will change the perceived patterns of quantum physics by using its alien offspring to bring into focus the phenomena of paranormal and spiritual experience.

Quantum Mechanics:
The Certainty of Uncertainty

In what follows, I will basically paraphrase and amplify the clearest general description of quantum physics that I've read so far. It was given by Steven Weinberg for the 1986 Dirac Memorial Lecture at Cambridge University and recorded, together with Richard P. Feynman's lecture for the same occasion, into a book called <u>Elementary Particles and the Laws of Physics</u>.[1] Of course, the commentary about parapsychology is my own.

Quantum mechanics, the mathematical arm of quantum physics, begins with probability theory. Probability theory is very simply based on a toss of the coin resulting in a heads or tails result. There is an equal chance of getting either one, so ideally in a hundred trials there would be 50 heads and 50 tails. A schematic diagram can show this as a graph with heads in the vertical direction and tails in the horizontal direction. This is a Newtonian kind of linear construct. However, quantum physics wants to know about and describe all the possibilities in between the two of heads or tails. Therefore, in quantum mechanics, the state of the coin cannot be described simply as heads or tails so it is called a state vector.

(See Figure 14., *State Vector*. The limits of the state vector is heads or tails, but the arrow of the state vector can point in innumerable directions going in between those two.)

If the coin is in the vector in which the arrow points in the diagram, then it is neither in the heads or the tails position. The arrow may be closer to the heads or closer to the tails position but only if it is clearly upright or horizontal will it be definitely in one or the other. Quantum mechanics regards all the other positions as definite possibilities, and here let me quote from Weinberg because it is too astounding to accept from a meddling, paranormal, spiritual, metaphysical, non-physicist. He says,

> "However, by looking at the coin you will force it into one of these two possibilities....When you measure whether the coin is heads or tails, it will jump into one configuration or the other with a probability that depends on the angle that the arrow had initially." (Weinberg 1987)

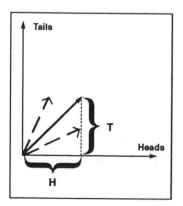

A coin as an example of a simple quantum mechanical system.

Figure 14.
State Vector

The limits of the state vector is heads or tails, but the arrow of the state vector can point in innumerable directions between those two.

So the closer the angle of the arrow is to heads or tails the more likely is it that it will wind up as either one. But it won't become either one until you look at it. In its intermediate state, there is no way of knowing just where it is. Then, by a physicist's acting upon it, it will leave its intermediate state and take the quantum leap into the either-or state needed for everyday reality. (We will reserve the question of whether humans other than physicists may act upon the arrow in its intermediate state to affect its outcome.)

All the rest of quantum mechanics is a mathematical working out of how and under what conditions the probabilities of the state vector will lead to heads or tails. In other words, how do you get from an essentially invisible, unpredictable and therefore unknown state of affairs to one that manifestly is visible, predictable and knowable was the dilemma initially posed by quantum physics. Though there are quite a few unresolved problems which concern us and which I will take up later, physicists have been extremely successful in predicting, experimenting on and performing this feat, within the context of quantum mechanics.

However, I have a problem with the fact that although Weinberg, among others, states that the fact of a person acting upon the state vector is what makes it jump into a heads or tails position, none of the theory or of the experimentation or of the mathematics actually includes the complex factor of the possible effect of the person looking at the coin. The real effect of the person that makes the coin jump from its probable state, from its state of tendencies, into its actual state which we call this or that, into everyday reality is ignored except theoretically. Von Neumann, as we saw earlier, was the only scientist who attempted to give the person a real place in the quantum leap and it was rejected. This lack of inclusion is what I think leaves a big hole in quantum physics' attempt to describe the whole nature of the universe, which is what Weinberg implies in calling his lecture: "Towards the Final Laws of Physics".

A Brief History of the Holes in Quantum Physics

It is necessary to review the subject of the history of quantum physics in order to see what are its constituent parts and to find out how this hole in its theory evolved. We will find out it actually has many holes, like swiss cheese.

Briefly, during the dominant period of Newtonian physics which began over three hundred years ago, all matter including light was considered made up of particles. There was a conflict between particle and wave proponents that goes back to 1690 when Christian Huygens proposed that light spread as waves in the same way as sound and water waves. However, Huygens was ignored because Newton's authority was so immense that the particle theory he favored held sway for another century until the Thomas Young experiment in 1803 (Pais 1991[2]). With Newton, particles were thought to be the basic component of the physical universe and everything known at the time followed from that premise. Newton's laws of motion and the verifiable mechanical operations that resulted from them established a scientifically predictable system in which particles, objective facts and repeatability, described in terms of mathematical operations, were the basics of a stable, scientifically determinable universe.

Then in 1803, one hundred and two years before Einstein published his work on relativity, Thomas Young performed his famous diffraction experiment which demonstrated that light was made up of waves, not particles, restoring Huygens' position, or so it was thought.

Throwing a pebble into water causes a wave front made up of highs and lows, crests and troughs. When two wave fronts meet in water, their interaction increases crests and troughs; if the crests meet they augment to become highs while the meeting of crest and trough will cancel each other out leaving the low part of the wave.

Young's experiment showed that the same effect occurs in interactions between light beams. Young sent a ray of light through a diffraction grating, a piece of solid material with two slits. He found that when light was going through only one of the two slits it showed up as a unitary shape (as when you shine a flashlight) on a screen; however, light going through both slits showed up, not as two shapes which you would expect from light if it were made up of particles, but as alternating light and dark bands equivalent to crests and troughs (looking like the light and dark bands venetian blinds might make on a wall).

(See Figure 15., *The Effects of Wave Interference.* The alternating light and dark bands are due to the effects of constructive and destructive wave interference, in just the same way that highs and lows come about in wave fronts in water.)

Light was therefore obviously made up of waves, it was thought, and not of particles, as Newton had supposed.

This conclusion was changed again in 1899 when Max Planck, to solve a mathematical problem in which it appeared there could be an infinite number of energy vibrations of radiant energy (the "Jean's box problem", in which "infinite" is an unusable number experimentally) coming out of a black box like a stove radiating light and heat, proposed the existence of a light quanta which would be the smallest possible package of energy that light could have. Light is not a wave, he said, nor is it the classical particle, but is composed of light quanta which are minimum individual packages of light energy (Gamow 1958 [3]) However, even though they appear in particle-like packet form, quanta are measured in terms of wave dynamics according to frequency and wave length, creating the particle-wave dilemma.

Accepting Planck's theory that light travels in the form of individual energy packets in space, Einstein added experimental evidence that when a quantum (as he called it) of light hits an electron it must transfer all its energy to the electron, compelling the electron to leave the atom, in what came to be called "The Photoelectric Effect".

Einstein's proposal that "light propagates through space in the form of individual energy packages, and ... on encountering an electron, such a light quantum communicates to the

a.

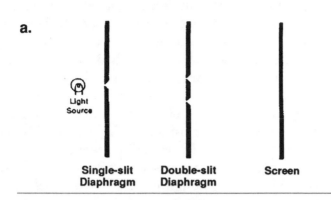

Single-slit	Double-slit	Screen
Diaphragm	Diaphragm	

The ability of light to diffract around corners and through small holes can be tested using a single slit to make a circular wave and a double slit to produce interference.

b.

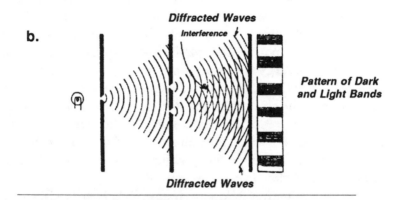

Like water ripples passing through a hole, the light waves spread out in circles from the first slit, moving "in step" with one another. Circular waves advancing from each of the holes in the doubly slitted screen interfere to produce a pattern of light and shade on the viewing screen — clear proof that, as far as this experiment is concerned, light behaves as a wave.

Figure 15.
The Effects of Wave Interference

The alternating light and dark bands are due to the effects of constructive and destructive wave interference.

electron its entire energy" only left physicists with further proof that the particle-wave dilemma was real. (Gamow, 1958, P. 295). This became evident in the fact that a light quantum, or a photon as it was later called, communicates to the electron its entire energy. But a quantum of light is measured as a wave while an electron is measured as a particle. How can there be an effect of one upon the other? It's as if when a baseball hits an orange, instead of missing it or smashing it the baseball turns into an orange.

Attempting to solve the particle-wave dilemma led to an expansion of quantum physics, providing it with much of its early developmental excitement. Bohr's discovery of the quantum rules that electrons move as discrete energy packets in an atomic nucleus threw out the assumptions of continuity in velocity followed by conventional Newtonian mechanics, and replaced them with the first set of rules for quantum mechanics, namely, that electrons follow restricted orbits and jump in unit amounts from orbit to orbit according to changes in energy states in neighboring orbits. The energy difference between the changes among those two states is emitted from the electron in the form of a Planck-Einsteinian light quantum. (Again, a light wave is the form of energy emitted when electron particles jump from one orbit to another, a conversion in form which is an energy radiation from electrons that can be measured.)

After the dilemma following upon Niels Bohr's discovery that, contrary to the continuity expected of relationships in Newtonian theory, there were discrete bands within which the electrons circulated, quantum theory was given an enormous research impetus. Rutherford was the first to respond to Bohr's new ideas as follows:

> "There appears to me one grave difficulty in your hypothesis, which I have no doubt you fully realize, namely how does an electron decide what frequency it is going to vibrate at when it passes from one stationary [discrete] state to the other? It seems to me that you have to assume that the

electron knows beforehand where it is going to
stop'. [Pais, the author, comments as follows:] In
typical Rutherford style he had gone right to the
heart of the matter raising the issue of cause and
effect, of causality: Bohr's theory leaves unanswered not only the question why there are discrete states but also why an individual electron
in a higher state chooses one particular lower
state to jump into. In 1917 Einstein would add a
related question: How does an individual light-
quantum, emitted in an atomic transition, know
in which direction to move [in the Photelectric
Effect]? These questions were to remain unresolved until...quantum mechanics gave the surprising answer: they are meaningless."
(Pais 1991)

The answer quantum mechanics gave that made the question meaningless was a series of mathematical formulae
which thereafter enabled scientists to predict, within the
Principle of Uncertainty, what quantitative characteristics
would result in what quantitative behavior on the part of
atoms with their constituent nuclei and electrons. Actually,
it ignored the questions asked by Rutherford and Einstein
because they managed to attain mathematical answers which
gave empirical and logical results. After that, the rest became
unimportant, therefore "meaningless".

How does the electron "know" what to do is, in essence,
however, part of a set of questions that repeatedly reappears
in various forms and never receives an adequate answer in
physics. The question of why it behaves as it does is not
answered just because the mathematical how of its behavior
is clarified. This is the hub of the dilemma, unanswerable
by physics, that enables us, indeed makes it absolutely
necessary to tie in quantum theory to the spokes of an
additional, non-mathematical explanation such as can be
found in quontic psychological theory. Another level of explanation was still needed.

The question of what and how the electron knows how to act is related to and is similar in a way to the dilemma inherent in paranormal phenomena. How does whatever may be the medium of communication between paranormal and material existence know that a transfer of energy is in the offing, where to go with that energy, and what vibratory frequency it should react with?

How can we integrate physics into a paranormal or metaphysical theory which includes the human factor when at this point in physics there is still no sense of the necessity of including real variables for a human observer at all?

A second unanswered question, or hole in the whole, comes from the interference experiment in which the electron seems to "know" whether it must go through one or two slits and behave like a particle or a wave without answering how it knows.

Another hole was created by the photoelectric effect experiment, changing baseballs into oranges, which made absolutely no Newtonian sense. The result was "irrational" and had to be explained, which was what Einstein set out to do. However, his additional experiments, in the conceptual sense, only made matters worse.

The diffraction experiment was conducted again, this time with a single photon shot first through one, then through both slits in the diffraction grating. Going through a single slit, the individual photon acted like a particle in the same way that an entire beam of photons would have done; and going through the double slit, the single photon acted like a wave with alternating light and dark bands appearing on the screen, showing an interference pattern. The single photon behaved as if it were minimally two photons by going through two slits simultaneously.

How can a single photon, choose, or know enough, to act like either a particle or a wave? Where does the option come from? What enabled it to respond to the different experimental situations appropriately? How could a photon (with no intelligence) appear to "understand" the situation in which there was either one or two slits and to make choices that were appropriate to the different experimental elements? In effect, it seemed able to split itself into two particles going through the double slit grating but remained one particle in the single slit grating.

Psychological Dilemmas

First, let us take up the question that was asked about how the electron or photon knows to behave like a particle or a wave, whether in multiples or singlets. Talbot suggests an answer held by some physicists:

> "The answer given by quantum physics is as astonishing as it is profound. It is that each photon somehow goes through both openings at the same time and thus carries some sort of knowledge of the status of both slits when it strikes the photograph. ...[Prior to striking the plate] it does not exist as a single object. During this phase it quite literally seems able to manifest as several probabilistic counterparts of itself and explores all possible pathways open to it simultaneously. It is only when it reaches the photographic plate and leaves a single point of impact that it appears to abandon its multiple existences and once again returns to behaving like a solitary projectile....This is why physicists speak of the wavelike phases of such particles not as material waves, but as waves of probability."
> (Talbot 1988 [4])

Probability and having knowledge means that choices are being offered and have to be made. All the conditions for such choices are certainly not known - if indeed this is an accurate description of what occurs. Nevertheless, it is worth examining some of the issues involved if making a choice is truly the dynamic of the photon's action.

The problem remains that choice among various possibilities also introduces the factor of consciousness. And for consciousness to exist there has to be input from memory. The dynamics of interaction between consciousness and the object of its input is not clear as yet, particularly when that object is an electron. Nevertheless, it is logically conceivable that the experimenter's consciousness might become a part of the outcome of any experiment. To stretch that possibility to its mystical limits, perhaps there is some kind of consciousness inherent in the photon, or better yet in all nature, as the Easterm mystics proclaim, and this universal consciousness is in correspondence with the consciousness of the experimenter. Certainly, if the entire universe is ultimately a composition of a unified network of forces, energies, and potentia with their interaction determining the resulting effects, then the experimenter himself must have a place in the equation. Thus the unifunctional mind assumes a position of relationship between metaphysical and human inputs. We will attempt to integrate physical and psychological issues further in what follows.

Psychology and the Particle-Wave Dilemma

In approaching the particle-wave dilemma from a psychological viewpoint we have a unique advantage and this is the advantage of analyzing data from an awareness of the power of consciousness as a guiding force, or energy, capable of affecting, influencing and participating as a part of matter. Consciousness, as seen in this presentation is also an ally of memory and homeostasis, functioning something like a nursemaid to humanity, watching over things to see that it all works out well. Consciousness has to give her baby room to move freely yet wants to see that he won't get hurt. To perform her job well consciousness has to know about certain kinds of things that affect her baby. Knowing about things also means having a memory about the way things are as well as awareness of what is best for her charge. In the interests of her charge's survival she must keep energies affecting him in a homeostatic state, protecting him from suddenly destructive forces.

Without pressing the analogy too hard, we have suggested that the particle-wave situation manifests something like a memory, and therefore memory, which functions along with homeostasis through consciousness, is guiding events everywhere. Memory, we have seen, is an essential ingredient in human consciousness but more than that it, along with homeostasis, seems essential to the constitution of our universe itself to provide it with stability and continuity.

For instance, whether an energy state takes the form of a particle or a wave might be due to the signalling of a memory state which, having accomplished this simple task an infinite number of times, knows exactly how to relate to it and a mnemonic energy is guiding it. There is a total atomic response being made to signals coming from the environmental situation which results in appropriate behavior in response to the limiting parameters it encounters.

Physicists, we have seen, do not regard an atom as an object with a definable material form. It is an energetic response, coming out of a sea of infinite events and therefore infinite possibilities (the "Dirac Sea" as it is called which we will discuss later) into a particlar form. The particularities of the form are evidently an outcome of the combination of "memories" available (in the quontic warehouse/Dirac Sea) from each of the elements contributing something to the outcome. For there to be an outcome at all, there must be a homeostatic-memory-survival axis on which the outcome turns.

The outcome is unifunctional in the true sense of the word in that the end result is a composition in which the parts are in some sense in touch with the whole. Even so, "the whole" for physics does not include anything paranormal or spiritual and, at the most, it only includes the experimenter in some physical sense as an observer who has set up the experimental situation in a practical way out of his desire to explore a particular aspect of a theory, but not as a conscious being whose specific energies may interact with the experiment to help define its results.

Of Quantum Physical Reality: A Review and Expansion

Let's return to the story of the particle-wave dilemma as it unfolded in physics, reviewing as we go. It is important to follow the history of the particle-wave dilemma because there are consequences which affect the broad outline of the quontic psychological theory we have proposed as well as leading to specific concepts which can influence our understandng of paranormal phenomena such as past life regression.

In 1923, Louis de Broglie suggested that since photons are measurable as waves, electron particles which are constituents of photons are actually waves and therefore all matter is made up of waves. A couple of years later, in 1925, Erwin Schrodinger developed a mathematical formula for De Broglie's observation called the probability wave equation (probability wave function) which has held its validity in every quantum equation, thus solving innumerable problems in quantum physics. It gives the probability that a wave will be observed as a particle. The Schrodinger formula led to quantum mechanics which is based on a mathematical formulation of matter as a probability wave. It states that the way we perceive matter, no matter how we experience it, is not an inevitable single fact of nature but is the result of an equation of probabilities which works out to become the one that we experience.

However well it solved many problems in quantum physics, the mathematical formulae of quantum mechanics also opened the door to a pandora's box of new problems. It closed one door, only to open many another dilemma. That is not unique and is clearly intrinsic to the process of scientific research. The effect of good research is to challenge and change the current point of view so that doors open to new research and further information points the way to further changes. All such research can not be included here so I will skip many significant experiments that are not so pertinent to our problem which is to relate physical theory developed in quantum mechanics to the broader functions of transpersonal experience.

Max Born was the physicist who, in 1926, observed that the probability wave function and quantum mechanics describe not matter itself but the likelihood of finding a particle in a particular place; therefore only the probability of an event, not the event and not matter itself could be described by the Schrodinger probability wave function. He pointed out that the wave function just says there is something acting beneath the event we call a wave which is described by a mathematical wave function through which we know that several possible events can exist. This idea led to the Many Worlds Interpretation by H. Everett in 1957, which was later advocated by such distinguished men as J.A. Wheeler, B. de Witt, and S. Hawking, and will also be amplified later, taken up in relation to the meta-physics of past life regression.

The probability wave function went in tandem with Heisenberg's Law of Indeterminacy. In Newtonian, three dimensional space, when a moving object is measured for location and speed it is possible to stipulate accurate measurements for each variable. However, it was discovered that describing the position and momentum of the electron in its orbit around the nucleus of an atom with accuracy for both measurements (position and momentum) simultaneously was impossible. If you determine how fast a particle is travelling, then its position can't be determined, and if you determine its position then its speed of travel can't be determined, except within an uncertain range. How the experiment is set up will determine which variable can be measured with accuracy, the other one is subject to uncertainty. This led to Heisenberg's Law of Indeterminacy (or Uncertainty) which states in mathematical terms how this inability to

determine both simultaneously operates. Taking the indeterminacy law a step further, the Copenhagen group offered
the interpretation that nothing at all can be said to exist until
an action is taken to determine its existence. The tree does
not fall in the forest if no one is there recording the fact of
anything having fallen. What is perceived is determined by
setting up the experimental situation and there is no objective universe prior to the experimental determination of its
existence. We live in an observer-created reality.

This would seem to be a real attempt to fill in one of the
holes in quantum mechanics, that is, to account for the effect
of the observer in the outcomes. However, the observer is only
included by the Copenhagen interpretation in a non-specific,
mechanical, abstract way. A mechanism with nothing but
a recording device for a mind would serve its purpose equally
well.

Something seems to have to trigger the electron to move
itself from an indeterminate state, or the state vector, from
its sitting on the fence of becoming (heads or tails) to push
it over into being (something). However, there was no
attempt to explain the factor of the trigger, and aside from
one rejected foray by Von Neumann into including consciousness as the trigger, nothing has ever been done by physicists
who remained in the physics mainstream to describe consciousness as a determining factor. Such an attempt to
include the human factor fully results in rejection or
displacement into a non-physics tributary of research.

The Copenhagen interpretation split the mainstream of
physics. Belief in an objectively given universe was threatened by the probability equation. The Copenhagen version
was dependent on an observer created reality — a quantum
transformation from a non-dimensional state with no prior
history into an actual state in three dimensions.

Einstein rose to meet the challenge which threatened his
belief in the existence of an objective universe. Einstein,
Podolsky and Rosen published a paper (Einstein et al. 1935[5])
called "The EPR Paradox" to counter the Copenhagen
interpretation's claim that the universe doesn't exist, in

effect, until an experimenter with his equipment enters it to do something to it or with it. The EPR experiment was a series of "thought steps" rather than an actual physical experiment which intended to show that the quantum interpretation was incomplete, that matter exists in its own right, that "God does not play dice with the universe" as probability theory would have us believe.

Local and Non-Local Causality

The EPR thought experiment was based on a conflict between relativity and the implications of quantum mechanics. The laws of Special Relativity limit the ultimate speed of anything in the universe to 186,000 miles per second and maintains that cause-effect relationships between objects are based on local, nearby, observable interactions. The EPR paradox intended to demonstrate that these hard and fast experimentally proven rules of physics would be violated by the expanded implications of quantum mechanics. The paradox intended to show that according to quantum mechanical rules, if it were correct, matter would demonstrably be influenced both non-locally and acausally, (on a quantum scale, a car moving in New York would affect a car in London) violating relativistic physical knowledge as well as common sense and therefore it was "incomplete". The results of the EPR paradox, however, gave out another message to their unconventional physicist colleagues. The EPR paradox had a powerful backlash.

In Newtonian physics and relativity, local causality determines how objects near each other affect each other's behavior according to Newtonian rules. If a person in a car turns on the throttle, puts it in gear and presses the gas pedal, the car moves. Neither the car in front, in back, or those in another city will move due to the driver's action. (We assume he's careful and doesn't bump into another car - but if he did, the bump itself making the second car move would provide another example of localized, cause and effect actions).

The EPR paradox intended to demonstrate that if quantum physics were correct it would imply the existence of a communication system which violated not only the rules of local causality in Newtonian physics, but it would imply the presence of some kind of "spooky action at a distance", as Einstein called it. By this he meant that a signal emanating in New York could be simultaneously apparent in London, if quantum mechanics were rigorously followed. If you start a quantum car in New York, that event will simultaneously start a quantum car in London. Such signals which defied the laws of local causality could also mean that something travelled faster than the speed of light, which also violated the Special Theory of Relativity's rule that nothing travels faster than the speed of light. Because it violated the classical rule of the determination of events through local causality and relativity theory, quantum theory was not adequate to describe the physical universe, according to EPR conclusions.

That started a spate of new experiments to disprove EPR's conclusions. J.S. Bell disproved it through the application of mathematics in quantum mechanics, creating The Inequality Theorem. Soon afterward, David Bohm and a French physicist named Alain Aspect demonstrated in two other experiments that an actually positive application of the EPR effect was real. The message given to physicists was that, contrary to what EPR intended, it could be demonstrated that particles are connected in a way that transcends our usual ideas about causality, at least on microcosmic levels.

Philosophic Implications:
Non-Local and Acausal Effects

In effect, what Bell's Inequality Theorem was able to show through quantum mathematics was that if locality existed by itself in classical and relativistic physics, then the three-dimensional world did not exist. He came up with the startling conclusion that reality must be based on non-locally determined events even on the three dimensional level or else quantum mechanics is wrong - and both these conclusions were impossible for most physicists to accept. Since using non-local interactions is the only way to adequately explain reality, then non-local interactions must exist or the world does not, according to Bell's Inequality Theorem. Bell's theorem did not necessarily indicate that the Copenhagen interpretation was correct or incorrect as much as it opened the door to the interpenetration of interactions among "quantum stuff" without the restrictions imposed by relativity and local causality.

This theorem has never been disproven, so it is tolerated by most physicists who still do not accept non-local causality but who totally accept quantum mechanics which is as fundamental to their understanding of reality as Newtonian theories are. (Although describing the EPR "experiment" and Bell's theorem in greater detail could be interesting, it would require an involved explanation regarding polarization and particle spin in paired electrons first as background. The amount of time necessary would be inappropriate for the purpose of this work. Both Herbert (1987) and Zukav (1984) provide succinct explanations.)

Bell showed that, at a basic, fundamental level, the parts of the universe are not separate but are interconnected in an intimate and intrinsic way. The "strange connectedness" that the EPR experiment should have disproven turned out to be even truer and more demonstrable than before, and reinforced with greater certainty the non-local "absurdity" that Einstein thought had been discarded.

Nevertheless, non-local communications is a phenomenon not easily proven or accepted in conventional science. The rejection of it is almost automatic despite its experimental demonstration. For instance, in a biological experiment, a phenomena whose synchronicity defied causal explanation occurred around the world, as reported by Sonea (1988[6]) Discussing the rapidity with which bacteria proliferated once they became adapted to "the miracle drugs" after the second world war, the author stated,

"...The most remarkable feature of these sudden resurgences of disease was that the bacteria that caused them simultaneously acquired, sometimes overnight, resistance to five or six antibiotics. Moreover, the resistance was worldwide; no sooner would a hospital in Tokyo report that a particular strain of Shigellae had stopped responding to tetracycline and streptomycin than would a clinic in San Francisco report the same. This baffled biologists, who believed bacteria acquired resistance through random mutation. But such a time-consuming process could not account for the speed with which the microorganisms had developed defenses against antibiotics."

However, the author found another explanation within the local causal rationale in an experiment which showed that genes called R plasmids are capable of replicating independently of the cells they occupy. He presumed that this would enable them to appear simultaneously with new resistant characteristics across the world. This has never been demonstrated, leaving it open as to how it was possible for a communication across the world to occur. Nevertheless, since R plasmids are a "real" causal type explanation, it was accepted. The alternative explanation would be that instantaneous and synchronous communication can occur in living cells whose communication system is acausal and therefore not dependent on locality or temporality, in the same way that Bell's theorem shows that atoms have that capability.

Reality as a Dependent Variable

In the mainstream of physics, Dirac, in the process of

developing the theory of quantum electrodynamics posited that the existence of an infinite sea of invisible, virtual, energy preceded the manifestation of energy in a particle form. Quantum physics is compelled to propose the existence of such a state, but is not able to resolve it into a measurement with a materialistic functional form. It takes a step into mysticism still too great for physics to understand that a functional form is not necessary for the existence of energy on every level.

Bell's theorem and Dirac's sea of virtual energy are close, also, to what the mystics have been saying all along; in effect, that the fabric of the world is one and indivisible. The world we think of as real is a projection of a larger reality and therefore it's an illusion to think that the material universe exists independently of a transcendant set of operations. Though neither Bell nor Dirac would agree with a mystical interpretation of the universe, they would agree that the universe is inconceivable without the presence of something like the "hidden variable" which is underneath observable phenomena, supporting and unifying the world of three dimensions.

Einstein, who favored a theory of objective, purely local reality even on the quantum level ultimately lost the battle to quantum mechanics which proved itself experimentally in every area it investigated. However, this acceptance did not necessarily include the philosophical implications of the hidden variable. The Copenhagen interpretation which declared that nothing existed prior to the functions brought into play by the manipulations of the experimenter served to make a hidden variable philosophically unnecessary.

However, neither the Copenhagen interpretation nor Bell's theorem finished the struggle to determine the nature of reality once and for all. Discussions and interpretations about the nature of reality bloomed like wildflowers in a field by a lake in the springtime, and they continue to proliferate. No one can lay claim to knowing the answer to what reality is all about. Indeed, it may turn out, as we will see later, that reality is not a set of actual facts at all but is a variable in a dynamical process which has many potentials. That reality could be a variable arising out of a hidden non-variable, out of a sea of quantum stuff or out of a fifth dimensional state, is not as unlikely as it first sounds, judging from quantum physical descriptions and explanations of its data.

For us, the question of probability in quantum physics has led to an additional question. Probability and the Bell Theorem imply that there are means of communications and options in the choice of form in material reality that are not always visible. Is there a relationship between the non-locality proposed in Bell's theorem, the atemporal possibility of signals that go faster than light speed and a situation like the diffraction grating experiment in which a particle can make a choice? If so, what does that allow us to infer about human processes?

To summarize the problem: this seems weird, that a particle or a wave may be able to choose its form by somehow assessing the situation within which it finds itself by means of a signal of a kind whose presence and dynamics we can't determine. How can the wave going through the single slit in the diffraction experiment turn into a particle, even if it "chooses" to do so? What kind of incredible information and communication process must be taking place?

Gribbin puts it this way:

> "What we see is what we get. An experimental observation is valid in the context of the experiment and can't be used to fill in details of things we do not observe. You might say that the double-slit experiment tells us that we are dealing with waves; equally, by looking only at the pattern on the detector screen you can deduce that the apparatus has two holes in it, not one. The whole thing is what matters—the apparatus, the electrons, and the observer are all part of the experiment....An electron leaves the gun and

arrives at the detector, and it seems to possess information about the whole experimental setup, including the observer....It is wholistic; the parts are in some sense in touch with the whole....The world seems to keep all its options, all its probabilities, open for as long as possible. The strangest thing about the standard Copenhagen interpretation is that it is the act of observing a system that forces it to select one of its options, which then becomes real." (Gribbon, 1984, P. 172) [7]

Doesn't this actually describe Reality as Variable in a total network of events more than as an invariant, objectively determining factor in shaping events? Up to now science has been treating "Reality" as an invariable determinant whose nature will determine the outcome of the experiment, and of life itself. However, the particle wave dilemma, the Copenhagen interpretation, and Bell's Theorem actually treat reality as a variable whose outcome depends on all the other inputs. Despite this, in actual scientific practice, reality continues to be treated as an invariable determinant which precludes the outcome, as if its rules need only be correctly assessed and assembled.

This perceptual difference is a crucial one for the psychic experiment in which the most important inputting factor relies on an outcome from the transpersonal experience and skill of the psychic person. The reality outcome is then dependent on the level of consciousness available to the person who desires to affect reality. Psychic healing and the practiced development of mental healing power is an example of "the psychic experiment" IN WHICH THE DEPENDENT VARIABLE IS REALITY. In transpersonal experience it is fundamental that reality is a variable whose representation is determined by non-objective energetic acts whose effects are difficult to prove with current scientific and mathematical methods.

Quontic Psychological Reality:
A General Integration

The basic dilemma that quantum theory still needs to resolve, from this point of view, is the lack of acceptance of the hidden variable as independent and reality as the dependent variable, both acceptable in fifth dimensional dynamics. It has still not been accepted in science because:

First, on the Newtonian three dimensional level, which is still the basic explanation for the mundane macrocosm, all phenomena have to be objectively, mechanistically and mathematically represented as formulations about the funamental nature of particles interacting with each other. However, on the level of quantum theory, "particles" are actually the outcome of waves of probability, and are not themselves objects even though in three dimensions they may behave as if they were. How do scientists explain their transformations between manifesting as a wave or particle on their detection equipment when, despite the successful mathematics of the Schrodinger equation, they don't know of a scientifically describable mechanism by which such a relationship of transformation can exist? They reject the question because the mathematics of wave mechanics works without the theoretical explanation. In rejecting the question, however, quantum mechanics leaves itself vulnerable to the EPR charge that it is incomplete. It doesn't satisfy because even though it has the mathematical explanations it doesn't deal with the wholistic issue of explaining its data in reality.

Secondly, another as yet unexplored possibility exists, which is unacceptable because it doesn't come out of a scientific laboratory. It is that energy is not a thing, intrinsically has no form, and itself has no intention to do anything. It (the Parenchyma) is guided by fifth dimensional dynamics such as the homeostatic principle. If it does anything at all, it simply responds to the information given to it, organizing matter according to the stipulations of homeostasis vis a vis the environment it finds itself in. It is also circumscribed in its action by the information it receives within its environment. In the particle-wave dilemma, one slit is one kind of information, two slits is another kind of information and the electron responds in a manner characteristic of itself. It has its own history of interacting with the information in a form of energy feedback provided by its targeted object in the environment. When this information is stored and affects behavior in any way it is information with energy that we call memory.

How the electron responds is a characteristic determined by itself in the context of its history with a response to energy received from its environment. However, we have previously suggested that the sources of energy to which matter responds is not just three/four-dimensional but includes a fifth dimension.

The electron must have a history of its own since it wasn't created in fact by the experimental set-up. It had a self-determining existence of its own prior to becoming a visible electron. It was only signalled and then was given information by the lab equipment which it then responded to according to its prior history. That history secondarily developed in the larger physical context of the earth, which developed a history in the context of the galaxy, which came out of the history of the Big Bang, or something else, and so on. If there is an objective factor here then it is an outcome of the context of the interplay of information gathered and stored by electrons. It is that history that leads the electron into its ensuing engagement in its path of activity in the visible world.

But even in physics there is a universe of activity prior to the materially definable one (which will be elaborated further in the ensuing chapters.) Sourcing that "meta-physical" (prior to becoming observable) level of information in any way by a human intermediary already alters the flow of information available in the material situation. The interplay of information between fifth and third dimensional energies cannot be available in its purely meta-physical form within a three-dimensional space, so it has to become translated and transposed in order to be understood. It has to be placed in a material and in a human context.

This is what is done more easily by studies of meta-physics than by scientists who can understand the dilemma but are so dependent on their purely physical operations that they become trapped within the dilemma. That is the dilemma created but not resolved by the Copenhagen interpretation and by the Schrodinger equation. They eliminate an unpredicable pre-existent universe in favor of a probable universe with tendencies and capabilities to do this or that, depending on what is provided at the level of measureable information input, and ignore the nature of their assumptions for the sake of the level of measured objectivity they can manage to attain.

The Schrodinger Cat dilemma is the quintessence of the unresolvability of this dilemma using nothing but quantum physics as the determinant of reality (Gribbin 1984). You will never know whether a quantum cat that you never saw was dead or alive before giving it poison. In fact, it could have been both in quantum theory, and is not determinable. In meta-physical perceptions, if you could not see it, it was neither dead nor alive but existed in another form which is not available to describe in "life and death", measured, objective terms.

Nevertheless, physicists, even those accepting the Copenhagen interpretation still think in terms of the conventional paradigm of three dimensional reality based entirely on objectively determinable events in rejecting parapsychological information. One of the purposes of the "Models of Consciousness" chapter was to show why it is so difficult to overcome the conventional paradigm: it is psychoneurologically imbedded in a developmental process that begins in childhood, and not in scientific college physics courses as physicists would like to think. There is neither blame nor judgement intended in that statement.

It was Niels Bohr's Copenhagen interpretation that offered a realistic looking stageset to quantum physics so that it could play out its role on the world's scientific scene with a believable philosophical basis in reality.:

> "The particle and the wave, he [Bohr] proposed, are related aspects of a single reality that cannot be fully observed from our limited perspective, because any experiment that illuminates one aspect of it inevitably interferes with the other. Thus, the only solution was to renounce a complete causal description of the phenomena of light. To make such a concession would 'appear' very deplorable' he allowed—causal description being the raison d'etre of science—but it was in fact the key to a better understanding of the world.
> ....The notion of complementarity serve(s) to symbolize the fundamental limitation...of our ingrained idea of phenomena as existing independently of the means by which they are observed." [8]

The Copenhagen interpretation thus states that we can only perceive those phenomena that we physically prepare ourselves to see and the dilemma arises that when we prepare to see one type of thing we block out the possibility of perceiving another aspect of that phenomenon. (How well they could apply this insight to themselves!) Unfortunately, our perception of reality is never complete because the means predisposes the ends so that one level blocks out the other.

The second still unresolved dilemma arising from quantum physics is to explain the transmission of "knowledge", or a communication that looks like knowledge, passing through and among electrons within the quantum environment in disregard of conventional local and causal relationships and of the speed of light. (Science News Feb. 11, 1989 [9]) Does this open the door to the possibility of faster then lightspeed signals in an atemporal, non-local environment? Quantum physics, in some ways an offshoot of relativity theory, rejects the possibility of faster than light communications.

In Quontic Psychology we examined the existence of a possible transformation and communication mechanism operating within the Quontic Loop. Such a communication process would have to be faster than the speed of light, 186,000 miles per second.

The characteristics of faster than light, non-local influences are as follows:

a. They are not mediated by energy fields or anything else which take time to cross.

b. They do not diminish with distance and are as potent a million miles away as an inch away.

c. They link up one location with another without crossing space, without decay and without delay.

d. The response time of interactions is superluminal, (FTL). (Herbert 1985 [10])

Although according to relativity the above set of circumstances cannot be fulfilled, David Bohm, then teaching at Cambridge University attempted to reconcile relativity which limits lightspeed, and quantum mechanics which opens the door to acausality without embracing it, with the possibility of faster than light communications. To do so, he had to conceive two separate modes of existence which he called the "implicate" and the "explicate" orders.

Holographic Theory

The fear that some scientists have is that if non-locality is the basic modus operandi of the universe then locality and causality in physics have to be relegated to a secondary place or to the dust bin in our understanding of how the universe functions. This possible outcome bothered David Bohm also who sought for a way to include both paradigms into one reality without minimizing either.

In his Holographic Theory Bohm proposed the presence of another level of existence called "the implicate order" in which non-local communication among electrons was possible via an energy state in which the "pilot wave" was the transmission agent. The idea of the "pilot wave", as nearly as I can gather, was first proposed in 1923 by John Slater, one of the first American physicists who had seriously studied quantum physics at Harvard.

Slater is quoted as saying:

> "'You know those difficulties about not knowing whether light is old-fashioned waves or Mr. Einstein's light particles...I had a really hopeful idea...I have both the waves and the particles, and the particles are sort of carried along by the waves, so that the particles go where the waves take them, instead of just shooting in straight lines, as other people assume'. [Pais comments:] Thus Slater held on both to particles and to waves, the latter being a sort of pilot field that monitors the motion of photons. It is...the function of the field to determine the paths of quanta, and to specify the probability that they will travel along these paths.' His vision blends continuity, the radiation field, with discontinuity, atomic transitions."(Pais 1991 [11])

("Atomic transitions" are the tendencies of electrons to maintain discrete orbits until an electron in a lower orbit for any reason leaves its place, leaving an empty space, which becomes filled by an electron from a higher level orbit.)

Slater, who went to Copenhagen, caught the attention of Bohr and his colleague Hendrick Kramers and together the three physicists (BKS) wrote a paper attempting to reconcile the particle-wave dilemma, basing it on Slater's idea. There is a statement about it in Pais which I will quote in its entirety because it is at the heart of our problem.

> "BKS begin by recalling that the exchange of energy and momentum between matter and radiation [recall the particle-wave dilemma and the photoelectric effect] claims essentially discontinuous features. These have even led to the introduction of light quanta...'They abandon light-quanta in their own paper, replacing this concept by a new one ...The atom, even before the process of transition between stationary states takes place is capable of communicating with distant atoms through a virtual radiation field', a field distinct from the conventional, real, radiation field. This virtual field, carried by the atoms in a given stationary state, **was supposed to know and carry all the possible transition frequencies.** [My underline.] Emission of light in an atomic transition [during the quantum jump from one stationary, discrete orbit into a lower one] is, BKS posited, not spontaneous but rather induced by the virtual fields by probability laws analagous to those which in Einstein's theory hold for induced transitions'. Accordingly, the atom is under no necessity of knowing what transitions it is going to make ahead of time.'

In effect, the virtual fields induce, or guide, electrons from one orbit into another, the electrons simply following whatever the induction process demands of them, without their particularly 'knowing' why they are doing it. The atom, therefore, is following a meta-physical guide called "the virtual field" which was supposed to have total knowledge relative to transition frequencies. To continue this quote:

"Does communication with a distant atom, the receipt of a light signal emitted by another atom even before transition takes place not violate causality? It does. We abandon any attempt at a causal connexion between the transition in distant atoms, and especially a direct application of the principles of conservation of energy and momentum, so characteristic of classical theories... Not only conservation of energy...but also conservation of momentum [reduce to] a statistical law." (Pais 1991 [12])

The quotation is important because it is not only the predecessor to what Bohm later called the Holographic Theory with its concept of the pilot wave, but has the seeds in it of Everett's Many Worlds Theory, which will be taken up in greater detail in a later chapter. It is also just about the first theory to abandon the notion of the inviolability of local causality and even reduces the conservation of energy law to a statistical effect. Finally it implies the existence of a metaphysical form of energy (the virtual field, also called the pilot wave) which guides the physical form of atomic energy in its journey.

That was a huge, quantum leap for a physicist and indeed, those same elements caused it to flounder and it was rejected, even with such a respected physicist as Bohr behind it. In addition, Schrodinger's equation appeared shortly afterward and gave physicists the mathematically and experimentally foolproof evidence they wanted to solve the particle-wave dilemma. The mysterious "virtual radiation field" which is supposed to know everything that the electron has to do and its noxious information which can violate relativity theory wasn't necessary.[13]

De Broglie, the Nobel Prize French physicist who was also instrumental in reconciling the particle wave duality to everyone's satisfaction had also played unsuccessfully with the pilot wave idea, proposing that it guided the electron in its path around the nucleus of the atom. In both (BKS and de Broglie) of these usages, the pilot wave (or the virtual radiation field) was antecedant and interacted with a function of a three dimensional particle universe in which the contradictory simultaneous presence of waves and particles interacting had to be reconciled. However, due to the contradictions in the pilot wave with classical theory and the exception it took to conservation and causality, it was rejected by Einstein and other physicists though it was accepted by Born, and, oddly enough, by Schrodinger, even though it had no place in his equations. A later experiment "disproved" the theory on flimsy grounds but it was sufficient to displace it from consideration by the mainstream.

Bohm did not conceive it possible to rule out conservation and causality either but he appreciated both the theory of the pilot wave, and the evidence of non-local causality. He therefore, in his Holographic Theory, found a way to formalize a disconnection between the two by including both in a single theory which had the effect of reconnecting them again. He returned local causality and conservation by proposing two orders of physical functioning, the "unfolded" which was essentially the three-dimensional universe and the "enfolded" which is similar to what we have called the fifth dimensional universe. In Bohm's holographic use, the pilot wave is a higher, fifth dimension function. It is a stable part of the "implicate", "enfolded" universe which has a direct effect on the three dimensional "explicate" or "unfolded" order. The particle and the wave are restored to an interactional duality under the influence of a signalling process with the particle visible in three dimensional reality and the pilot wave functioning on the higher invisible level under non-local, a-causal rules.

> "The pilot wave, acting as a sort of probe of the environment, changes its shape instantly whenever a change occurs anywhere in the world. In turn, pilot wave communicates news of this change to electron, which alters its position and momen-

tum. When you make one kind of measurement, the pilot wave has one form; when you make another kind of measurement the electron takes on different attributes, because its pilot wave is different." (Herbert P. 49)

In Bohm's formulation, the pilot wave takes on a faster than light communication function that only was suggested but not developed by BKS.

Scientifically, neither the holographic theory nor Bell's inequality theorem settle anything at all for quantum physics except to challenge the old paradigms and cause a flurry of new experiments, but phenomenologically Bell and Bohm together do give paranormal psychologists theoretical fuel for their concepts.

Why not simply accept the Holographic Theory instead of creating the Quontic model? For one thing, the base of the holographic theory is physics whereas the basis of quontics, the questions that are explored, are resident in the modus operandi of the human organism, in the totality of its psychophysiology. This ultimately does include the knowledge gained through physics but is not where its priority lies. Quontic Psychology has a better psychological grandfather in the idea of Jungian Synchronicity which states that human behavior has both higher and mundane causes and levels of interaction; a domain of acausal, non-local communication may coexist that may influence and conjointly concur with events on the causal and local three dimensional plane in the human experience. The two planes are separate in their attributes, but there is some way in which they interact. How do they communicate with each other? Synchronicity and holographic theory are very similar in their explanations, but neither offers totally adequate solutions to this question of how the mind and matter levels communicate with one another.

The Pilot Wave is a good idea, and coming from a physicist gives it a scientific aura, but it opens up more problems than it solves. It tells us what it does, but not how it does it. The

Figure 16.   **Quontic Psychology**

Summary of Particle — Wave Dilemma

1665   Isaac Newton — All matter is composed of particles.

1803   Thomas Young — Electrons and light are composed of electromagnetic waves, not particles.

1905   Albert Einstein — Light is a quantum energy packet, a photon, a wave made up out of partilces bundled together.

1923   Louis de Broglie — Since photons are like waves, electron particles are waves and therefore matter is composed of waves.

1925   Erwin Schrodinger — Turned de Broglie concept into the probability wave question equation and created quantum mechanics, a mathematical formulation of matter as a probability wave.

1926   Max Born — The probability wave function describes not matter itself, but the likelihood of finding a particle in a particular place, the probability of an event, not the event and not matter itself.

1927   Albert Einstein — God does not play dice with the universe, the EPR paradox shows that quantum theory is not sufficient or complete, therefore probability theory is not accurate.

1927   Werner Heisenberg — The larger an object is, the less the magnitude of uncertainty in attempting to define momentum and position of a particle, the Uncertainty Principle. It is impossible to determine both position and velocity with perfect accuracy simultaneously. At the size of an atom, the uncertainty about one or the other is enormous.

1927   Niels Bohr — Principle of Complementarity establishes that particle and wave are complementary (like Yin and Yang). Which one is percieved is determined by setting up the experiment to see one or the other.

1927   Copenhagen interpretation — Nothing can be said to exist until an action is taken to determine its existence. Even then, whatever is "determined" is probabalistic, not certain. We live in an observer-created reality.

1927   Paul Dirac — Electromagnetic Field Theory and Quantum Mechanics integrated into a theory of quantum electrodynamics, the Quantum Field Theory. Results in discovery of anti-matter, the positron.

phenomena we are examining have had a lot of the "what" and too little of the "how" in their explanations. We will continue the story of developments in quantum physics to examine whether and how they may apply to quontic psychology in the next chapter.

The previous page, Figure 16., *Summary of Particle-Wave.*, shows the enormous explosion of research that took place between 1923 and 1927, years that culminated in the firm establishment of quantum physics as the new paradigm for atomic research.

The Purple Cow Dilemma

"Dismissing the unexplained...robs physics of much of its beauty. For physics, at bottom, is a wild, messy, unpredictable, eminently human business, full of strange accidents, inexplicable exceptions and weird, unrepeatable results—a science that thrives on anomaly, inconsistency and doubt. Certainty kills it."

— Hans Christian von Baeyer [1]

"When I examine myself and my methods of thought I come to the conclusion that the gift of fantasy has meant more to me than my talent for absorbing positive knowledge."

— Albert Einstein [2]

> I never saw a purple cow,
> I never hope to see one
> And I can tell you anyhow,
> I'd rather see than be one.

— Unknown

Those Regular White Cows

Well, we know what color cows are, the sacred kind that is, and they are not purple, they are conventional white. Maybe some have black markings. That's O.K. because some physicists, particularly J.S. Bell and David Bohm have begun to say there might be purple cows out there somewhere too. Of course, paranormal people are seeing them everywhere all the time, and some purple cows might even moo.

There's a little anecdote connected with the purple cow poem. Though many people I recited it to seem to have heard it before, I heard it audibly "spontaneously" for the first time at the moment that I wrote about "Spooky action at a distance", describing Einstein's EPR experiment in the last chapter. At first I was completely confused as to its source since I couldn't find any objective auditory stimulus. Was I hallucinating hearing it? After due investigation I found that the poem came unbidden over my little battery operated travel radio sitting on top of my computer. I did not turn it on and it had never before behaved in this way in the four years or so that I'd owned it. Neither has anything similar recurred in the four or five years since this incident took place. The suggestion is obvious that this was a beautiful case of synchronicity with spooky action at a distance demanding attention and confirmation. In addition, the poem had come on during a program instructing people how to improve their memory, and I could not turn the radio off without removing the batteries. The poem's timing was too wonderfully appropriate to ignore so I included it here. For me, the purple cow is not only visible, it audibly roars.

What has become very apparent as I've continued to study physics through books written by professionals and laymen is that physics is not a science without a bias. Physicists tend to be adament about the objectivity of their science, but within that statement lies a need to prove a theory at all cost, even at the cost of truly impartial demonstration of the objective facts, if there is indeed such a thing.

Unfortunately I have little actual interest in higher mathematics, but I get the distinct impression that mathematics itself, far from being a purely objective manifestation of what is, itself can be a way of manipulating data to explain the objects it describes in such a way that they will be shown to perform in the way that the scientist prefers. In the structure of how he conceives the rules of the game the physicist makes certain moves which will accomplish winning goals. The Copenhagen Interpretation was clearly based on a similar premise, viz: that you get the kind of results that are prescribed by the way you set up your experimental apparatus, particularly in the particle-wave dilemma discussed in the last chapter. It is important to recognize that uncertainty may not only be due to how you set up an experiment but whether you have a bias that requires a particular goal to be achieved. That's one reason why theories are often so controversial and many of them fall by the wayside, only to become resurrected at a later date with data in their favor.

Why is that important for us? Because the rejection and denial of data that does not fit in with the preconceptions of physicists who need to "prove" that certain things exist in the real world needs to be corrected in science. Only when the method of proof is corrected to truly include all the data "objectively", that is, without prejudice, will the data about psychological and psychic experience receive their just place in a scientific paradigm.

The Metaphysical Empiricists

As I traced the course of modern physics, I found a very interesting thing happened. Sometime after 1927 when Paul Dirac published mathematical formulae that led to quantum field theory, a split developed in the ranks of physicists. One group remained true to the rational, logical notion that facts that you can prove through experimentation in "the real world" and which can be expressed mathematically and therefore objectively are the only facts that belong in the physical sciences. This group rejected the possibility of there being an ether or any other medium in the "vacuum of space" which might act as a carrier wave for energy after the Michaelson-Morley experiment "proved" empirically that the ether did not exist; they also wrestled with mathematical infinities that continually reappeared in quantum physics experiments, attempting to "renormalize" these apparently aberrant results. They had equal difficulty with "zero energy" and "self-energy", concepts which introduced negative energy states into positive energy physics, (which we will look at more carefully soon) that is, states characterized by less than zero energy or infinite energy in readout, a condition which logically could not exist in a world that was made up of visible, finite, empirical, measureable matter only.

Perhaps, "split" is not the right word since there had always been metaphysical scientists ever since the alchemists who looked at non-physical phenomena as a way to better understand physical phenomena. Perhaps "it gained impetus" would be a better way to put the division between the pragmatic empiricists and the metaphysical empiricists. Both groups can be called empiricists because they regard experimentation as a fundamental means of exploring and arbitrating questions of reality. However, they seem, compulsively, to arrive at completely opposed interpretations of the same data.

The Business of Science

There is a somewhat acknowledged behind-the-scenes power-driven manipulation and misrepresentation of data in the scientific establishment, just as there is in any other moneyed, monopolized American industry. The leaders in the sciences have built up their corporations (academic as well as governmental and industrial), have cultivated and managed the rules operating in their companies carefully and will not allow anyone to get the benefits of the game who doesn't follow their rules very closely. The interpretation that becomes the accepted model therefore has a certain amount of social-economic factors built into it, such as prestige and large grant monies from government, industry and academia.

This is a judgement about the simple truth that it is not possible for anyone in Western society to function successfully in this, or any culture for that matter, unless they have adapted to socially developed biases. It is inevitable that some socially accepted preferences become a modus operandi in society. Witness the fact that perhaps the exceptions to this general rule are those in severely disturbed mental states who have no sense of personal preferences and possible choices, who see innumerable possibilities and therefore are unable to function on the basis of their preferences and run in circles trying to make decisions. On the opposite end of this continuum are those who are "experts". Whenever they talk about anything, they are fearful they might be seen as doubtful or wrong in making up their minds. Certainly there are courageous exceptions to this point of view: people who aren't concerned about being right or wrong but for whom the value of accumulating empirically personal and truthful experience is what counts.

David Bohm is perhaps the most recent renowned theoretical physicist to break with the pragmatic group after having successfully developed and been recognized for theories based on his empirical experience in physics. He was preceded by many less known experimenters in other fields such as Nicholas Tesla in electrical engineering, Wilhelm Reich in psychotherapy, Semyon Kirlian and Viktor Adamenko who were scientists in the Soviets, and the group which met at the Prague Conference in 1973 which led directly to what is today called Psychotronics.

As an interesting aside, for a definition of Psychotronics, I quote from the Jan-Apr. 1989 Newsletter of the New York Psychotronics Association - Chapter of USPA, (for which I served as editor at that time) as follows:

"Psychotronics, comes from two roots: *psycho* meaning mind and *tronics* meaning science. Psychotronics is, therefore, a mind-science. It is defined as the science of the interrelationships

> between mind, body and environment. It is,
> therefore, an interdisciplinary science concerned
> with matter, energy and consciousness....By add-
> ing the Mind-Matter interaction to our conven-
> tional sciences (where it is traditionally avoided),
> psychotronics derives an expanded science which
> can deal not only with normal phenomena...but
> can also deal with paranormal phenomena. Thus,
> psychotronics becomes a bridge between physics
> and metaphysics...which attempt(s) to deal with
> and interrelate the hard sciences with the eso-
> teric sciences."

There are currently an increasing number of associations
which are able to include psychic healing as well as paranormal
phenomena into their definition of some variety of science
and this trend has become a potent international movement
with a growing body of adherents. The strange fact exists
that this movement often has taken its concepts from the
rejected ideas of the hard science of physics.

In this chapter we will examine what the pragmatic physicists discovered and trashed by calling them "impossible
conclusions". What is especially intriguing in quantum
physics is the breakdown of the empirical, objective, local,
cause and effect framework for legitimate scientific operations into a relativistic, non-local, probabilistic framework for
the pursuit of experiments. What traditional physicists still
share in common is the fear of data that, for some reason,
cannot be made visible and measured, or at least shows
promise of measurement, on current equipment and/or in
mathematical formulae.

There are many other sources of energy that might affect
the outcome of an experiment in physics and in other sciences
- other than the mechanically measureable ones (Becker
1985[3], Gerber 1988[4], Redner 1991[5]). Below are several
blatant examples of distortion based on the biases of physicists.

Two Cases of "Research Without Bias"

A scientist who doesn't follow the rules is Robert O. Becker. He is an M.D. who became interested in the body's self-healing capabilities while examining electromagnetic processes. In the course of his experimental work which showed that the body did indeed manifest self-healing responses to electromagnetic stimulation, he became concerned about low level radiation from electric power and telephone lines. He reports that after his experiments showed detrimental and destructive effects such as cancer, other scientists began criticising and losing interest in his work and ultimately he lost government grants as well as his government job. Becker had committed the heresy of challenging the government/industrial/utility company complex in the public interest. In 1979, a groundbreaking epidemiological study by Nancy Wertheimer showed that leukemia was more prevalent among people, and particularly children, living near power lines. Additional studies have sometimes reinforced and sometimes rejected the evidence for a connection between power lines and cancer (Ezzell 1991 [6]). In 1991 the issue took the form of battle lines drawn up between those most concerned about public health and those in government concerned about the income of the utility companies. Now, in 1993, only after the death of a child attributed to power lines near a school and a study in Sweden that showed a higher incidence of cancer among children living or going to school near power lines, the utility companies have finally joined the investigation.

Another example of a different type comes from the U.S. Psychotronics Association's newsletter of Sept. 1988 which carried an interesting article that applies to the conflicting choices about following the rules made by hard core scientists and avant garde researchers. The article quoted here was originally written by Paul Raeburn, AP Science Editor, and though the source for the newsletter article was the June 30, 1988 issue of the Erie Daily Times, the news item's origin was New York. It said, as follows:

"Researchers at five separate laboratories in France, Canada, Israel and Italy reported...they have identified a curious antibody reaction involving human blood cells that should, by any imaginable theory, be impossible....The researchers have found that antibodies that react with certain blood cells will continue to react when diluted far beyond the point where they should theoretically be able to."

Evidently, at extreme dilutions there are no antibodies left in the solution for blood cells to react to, yet they do respond as if there were antibodies present in the extremely diluted solution. The report of the reaction first appeared in Nature, the prestigious British science journal which is also notorious for its pre-emptive opinions which guard the scientific establishment from invaders. The editors of that journal did not believe the result could have happened but published the research findings anyway because they couldn't find anything wrong with the way the experiment was conducted, and the experimenters themselves were highly accredited. In fact, Nature's editors went so far as to take the unusual step of publishing an "editorial reservation" to inform their readers of their lack of support for the incredible findings.

The original discovery was made by Dr. Jacques Benveniste head of INSERM, a prestigious French medical institute, while attempting to develop a new blood test to identify allergies. Subsequently, the results were duplicated by two groups in Israel and one in Milan. In Nature's reservation, they stated, "There is no physical basis for such an activity. With the kind collaboration of Professor Benveniste, Nature has...arranged for independent investigators to observe repetitions of the experiments."

The findings have a bearing on the treatments given by doctors using homeopathic remedies to treat disease. Homeopathic treatment requires the use by the patient of the same toxic substance that causes a disease in a highly diluted form in order to cure or improve a disease and its symptoms. If Benveniste's findings are correct, they support the medically rejected homeopathic forms of treatment.

The later findings carried out under Nature's auspices were negative in three out of four attempts to duplicate the reaction. On that basis they totally rejected the original results, also rejecting and questioning the validity of their single positive finding. That austere scientific body came to those conclusions even though, in total, six out of all nine experiments came out in favor of the "impossible conclusions", well above the number the laws of probability and chance requires. In rejecting the positive conclusions of the affirmative experiments they rejected the scientific method which they claim to espouse. It's hardly a case manifesting scientific objectivity.

A second, more subtle issue, is the question of how one of the four experiments reported in Nature came up with positive affirmation while the other three produced negative results. Do we have here another example of the effect of the unconscious predisposition of the experimenters exerting an influence in the results? Probably, no amount of interviewing or research currently possible would resolve this question to anyone's satisfaction because the prejudices involved are themselves so intense as to affect any interviews or research that would be undertaken.

In our view, the argument is a variation on the local, causal vs non-local, acausal arguments in the EPR and Bell theories. What is the basis of communication in living, and non-living, matter? Is it purely local and physically three dimensional or does it transcend locality and obvious causality?

Another case involves the U.S. government's attitude toward psychical research. In early 1988 the National Academy of Sciences organized a body of "objective" scientists under the National Research Council to examine the results of paranormal research. The purpose was to determine scientifically whether the body of findings produced by the paranormal research community had any validity. The final report was again basically negative, debunking parapsychology as having "no scientific justification".

The American Society for Psychical Research issued a report evaluating the NRC findings which they published in brief in their July 1988 Newsletter. Looking more closely at the panel of experts, it found that the two principal NRC investigators had previous reputations for being predisposed against paranormal phenomena. None of the panel members was chosen from the groups of researchers who espoused and supported paranormal findings. Indeed findings that were favorable to parapsychology were selectively omitted from the report. And, despite their promise to do so, the panel could not produce alternative explanations for the anomalies in behavior which were explained parapsychologically. The ASPR challenge ends by strongly calling for "the identification of underlying mechanisms and the development of theoretical models" to provide adequate understanding of psi phenomena.

I cite this NRC report as another gross example of "impossible conclusions" which function simply to guard the status and perogatives of the ruling "junta" made up of scientists who violate their own rules of research when it would otherwise be necessary to admit the existence of phenomena explained by parapsychology which traditional science has failed to explain.

We shall soon see how physicists provide the same disservice to their science when they have produced major experimental evidence in physics that they proceed to discard or rationalize because it simply cannot be explained by means of conventional experimental logic.

The Nobel Prize for Infinity

I promised we would take a closer look at concepts in quantum mechanics which have been rejected by physicists even though these theories were valid results gained through their own experimental processes. As we have seen, a major force for both the discovery and the rejection of "impossible" results has been the Nobel prize winning physicist Paul (P.A.M.) Dirac. They are worth examining for the explanations they offer in studying the transpersonal domain.

Dirac, in 1927, worked on the integration of quantum mechanics and electromagnetic field theory. Soon after, Tomononga of Tokyo U., Schwinger at Harvard U. and Feynman at Cal Tech developed it further, making it an effective and accepted quantum field theory called quantum electrodynamics, or QED for short. Following is a brief summary of QED.

In physics, the pattern created by an iron magnet on iron filings illustrates the magnet's field; thus the pattern of the iron filings is the figure that reveals the strength and direction of the magnetic field in which it appears, however the field itself is not visible. Similarly, light is a pattern of quantum particles, called photons since Einstein's discovery, which illustrates the unseen presence of electric and magnetic fields (electromagnetism which James Clerk Maxwell demonstrated in 1861). Light of all kinds, infrared beams, radar waves and x-rays are forms of electromagnetic radiation. Photons are the carrier instruments that carry out the "policies" of an electromagnetic field. The problem of relating electromagnetic radiation (the field effect of electromagnetism) to matter in general, and on a larger scale how to reconcile the basic principles of quantum theory and relativity with electromagnetism, became the challenge that Dirac took up.

One of the problems in relating relativity and electromagnetic radiation on the quantum level is the enormous differences in scale between relative and quantum phenomena. The quantum scale occurs mostly around the Comptom wavelength of an electron which is about 4×10^{-11} centimetres which comes out to 40 millionths of a millionth of a centimetre. Relativistic distances have been measured in terms of the speed of light in millions of light years. However, atoms and photons are both surrounded by electromagnetic fields just as are the planets so there obviously had to be some way to relate the two or physics could not finally explain the world in which we live.

Renormalization, a way to wipe out infinities that crop up in equations, was an important part of the history of QED because infinities in mathematics were in the way of developing an empirical theory. Infinity can't be tested or measured by either calculations or devices. Dirac and Feynman in particular demonstrated how it was possible to get rid of the infinities so as to produce a renormalized, relativized quantum theory. That the Dirac equation was the first relativistic treatment of the electron doesn't say much to the non-physicist, except that the goal was accomplished by Dirac's mathematics.

He was able to show how, mathematically, the atom, the electromagnetic field and their interaction could be described and relativized. (He was thus able to prove a law that Einstein had discovered. It gave the probability that a given atom in a given state in a particular field, manifesting a particular configuration, would release or absorb a photon.) His equations related matter (the atom) to a field (wave) condition in which the matter of an electron was represented not as a thing-in-itself but became an energy-thing in relation to the effects of an invisible-thing (its energy field). It showed that matter is only matter when there is an electromagnetic field in which it can exist (another variation of $E=MC^2$). Although invisible, the electromagnetic field is an energy force in its own right reflecting and affecting any matter in its vicinity, and their interaction is reciprocal.

The mathematical niceties of the theory gave rise to a many-headed hydra which necessitated a change in the perception of the relationship between space, matter and wave energetics. As related in The Second Creation (Crease & Mann 1986[7]):

"As a step to quantizing [defining it in terms of energy bundles and trying to make it conform with Heisenberg's Law of Indeterminacy] the electromagnetic field, Dirac hypothesized that his harmonic oscillators transmitting energy waves did not disappear when there was no field evident. Rather, they went into a 'zero state' [of energy oscillation], in which they existed but could not be detected. Thus energy and its matter-thing could be existing in a non-measureable state as a result of Dirac's equations. Associated with the zero state oscillators were zero state photons; these, too, could not be detected....His mathematical scheme implied that empty space should contain billions of invisible photons ...."

— in a field that could not be measured. Following is a simpler description of the same phenomenon from Gamow (1958 P. 314):

"...Dirac came to the conclusion that, apart from the *ordinary* electrons which rotate around atomic nuclei or fly through vacuum tubes, there must also exist an incalculable multitude of *extraordinary* electrons distributed uniformly throughout what one usually calls empty space. Although, according to Dirac's views, each unit volume of vacuum is packed to capacity with these *extraordinary* electrons, their presence escapes any possible experimental detection. The *ordinary* electrons studied by physicists and utilized by radio engineers are those few excess particles that ...[are caused by] an *overflow* of *Dirac's ocean*, which is formed by the *extraordinary* particles, and they [the ordinary ones] thus can be observed individually. If there is no such *overflow* nothing can be observed, and we call the space empty."

Empty space with nothing apparently in it is therefore not empty, its contents are simply not visible or evident because certain conditions of appearance, or manifestation, or perception, have not been met. "Dirac's ocean", full of extraordinary electrons surrounds us on all sides, but because it is uniform and frictionless it is not palpable to our senses. Since it is not tangible, does it exist except in theory?

Without acknowledgement from Science, I think that the line between metaphysical and scientific theory has just about disappeared. Dirac's ocean seems no different than the unseen universe of the fifth dimension or from the metaphysical speculation of the everything that exists in nothing in Hinduism.

The next step is typical of the pragmatic physicist's ability to totally dismiss perhaps ninety percent of the structure of the universe because it doesn't fit in with experimental procedure. Dirac was able to state that as long as they (the invisible photons) didn't show up, their presence made no difference. However this dismissal of the "unreal" elements in their mathematics didn't last. "...When Dirac's theory was interpreted in light of the uncertainty principle, it turned out that in some sense the zero state photons **do** show up...."

Indeed, in 1931, an American physicist, Carl Anderson, presented confirmation that particles with negative mass do in fact exist. Furthermore:

> "As Einstein's equation $E=mc^2$ demonstrated, mass and energy are two forms of the same thing. Thus the uncertainty principle dictates that if any small area can contain undetectable energy, then, according to Einstein's equation, it can contain undetectable matter. This basic uncertainty is not just a lacuna in our knowledge. Mathematically, there is no difference between

this uncertainty and actual random fluctuations
in the energy (or matter) measured. Therefore,
at least in theory, because any space **might**
harbor particles for a short time, it **must** do so.....

"As strained through the uncertainty principle,
quantum field theory exposed a frightful chaos
on the lowest order of matter. The spaces around
and within atoms, previously thought to be empty,
were now supposed to be filled with a boiling soup
of ghostly particles. From the perspective of
quantum field theory, the vacuum contains random eddies in space-time: tidal whirlpools that
occasionally hurl up bits of matter, only to suck
them down again. Like the strange virtual images produced by lenses, these particles are
present, but out of sight; they have been named
virtual particles. Far from being an anomaly,
virtual particles are a central feature of quantum
field theory...." (Crease & Mann 1986)

However, Dirac was annoyed that the field of matter was
not sufficiently consistent with relativity which relates to
objective light, energy and matter only, not to a hypothetical,
virtual matter, light and energy. Attempting to solve this
problem led him eventually to come up with a revolutionary
new equation to describe an electron travelling through space
having four components, two associated with their spin and
two with particle energy.

Virtual particles could never be seen, but had real effects,
as it turned out. The first virtual particle was the positron.
It is described as the energy resulting from the existence of
a "hole" in the Dirac energy ocean. (Another hole in quantum
theory!) A positron is an electron with positive energy because in an ocean of invisible negative electrons a "missing
electron", having emerged into the empirical world, would
leave a space which would be its opposite, a positive energy
electron, or positron, also called the anti-electron and anti-

matter. In Crease & Mann there is the following account of Dirac discussing this issue at the Seventh Solvay Conference:

> "Dirac asked his audience to consider an electron floating through empty space-or, rather, not-so-empty space. At any given moment, the particle is surrounded by a swarm of virtual photons, electrons, and positrons, buzzing like ghostly bees around the particle in its progress. In the brief moment of their existence, the virtual positrons, which are positively charged, are pulled toward the real electron [negatively charged]; the virtual electrons are in the meantime repelled by the negative energy charges in the electron. The result is that the electron has a cloak of positrons; it is surrounded by a shimmer of ghostly antimatter. As the distance becomes shorter, the number of virtual particles grows, in accord with the uncertainty principle [that there is an inverse relation between determining the probable position and speed of a particle]. The result is that extremely close to the electron, its charge is blanketed by an ever-increasing, indeed endless snarl of virtual positrons. Dirac called the process of attracting virtual positrons and repelling virtual electrons the "polarization" of the vacuum, [and since the number of possible virtual electrons and positrons were infinite] it was yet **another** infinity in quantum electrodynamics." (Crease & Mann P. 99)

The authors continue,

> "According to Dirac's theory, an electron is not localized in a particular place, but has a set of probable locations that are scattered around a point of maximum probability like the cluster of holes around the bull's eye of a sharpshooter's

target. Moreover, these locations circulate around the center as if the target were spinning; according to Dirac's equation, this motion [around the target] is the spin of the electron. Lorentz had envisioned a little ball rotating when he calculated the electron spin velocity, and found that <u>it</u> <u>turned faster than the speed of light - a flat</u> <u>impossibility.</u>" [My underline.]

By using the average of the cluster of the radius of probable locations of the electron, and by making it a hundred times bigger than the electron envisioned by Lorentz, Dirac was able to make the velocity of spin slow enough to remove the conflict with relativity (which states that nothing can move faster than the speed of light) and to predict the strength of the spin. This enormous electron is then a statistical average, a hypothetical electron made up out of numerous hypothetical locations, constructed by Dirac for the sake of avoiding the faster than the speed of light result obtained by Lorentz for the electron's spin.

Dirac's new equation, however, was effective in producing explanations for experiments like the collision of two electrons, and it was thought that physics now explained just about everything. There was no longer any need to deal with infinities (which would imply the existence of an unmeasureable infinite space-time).

However, Nature moves in elusive ways. It wasn't to be so.

More Impossible Equations

The problems of negative energy can be expressed as follows: It turned out that the Dirac sea of electrons, when applied to Einstein's law of the equivalence of mass and energy, $E=MC_2$ also must be solved as $M=EC_2$. It implies the existence of negative mass - which was considered an absurd impossibility. A something with a no-mass quantity was not possible.

Ordinarily physicists would assume that the world had started off with all electrons in measureable, positive energy states, in which they would remain, and no harm would come from the theoretical existence of negative energy. However, negative or invisible energy states refused to remain entirely theoretical. The mathematical description of the theory and Einstein's relativity theory began to insist on the existence of negative mass - impossible since it could not be measured and everyone knew that mass can only be called mass when it can be detected, recorded and measured.

The problem was that an ordinary energy electron should be able to emit a photon, a bundle of energy in the form of light. The electron thereby changes its balance of negative and positive electron particles by having lost a photon, with only enough energy remaining to drop into a negative, or minus energy state. In fact, the mathematics of it requires that **most** electrons should end up with negative energy, and, as we've seen, negative energy necessarily implies negative mass. (Crease & Mann P. 86)

Now there is an ugly kettle of fish for any pragmatic physicist. Try as they might they could not get their equations and their theories out of the never-never land of an irrational, unseen, unmeasureable universe. Negative energy and negative mass, postulates about unseen and unmeasurable energies, all came from an equation that was developed to solve the dilemma that there was spin velocity that was faster than the speed of light (Lorentz's equation). That idea was unacceptable to relativity in the first place because it implied an infinite space-time. Dirac solved that one and now they had to contend with another impossible dilemma involving infinite energies.

Looking Closely at Nothing

Lorentz's equation had postulated the necessity of a violation of relativity's speed of light limitation of 186,000 m.p.s.. Dirac successfully slowed the velocity down to less than the speed of light but then found himself stuck with a kind of excess energy that could not be accounted for except as a form of negative energy, which itself could not be seen or measured. A negative energy state means that neither this kind of energy nor this kind of mass could be included in the logical pragmatism of physics to help formulate equations about "the real world". Either he had to accept a violation of relativity through Lorentz's equation or take a descent into negative energy which did not exist. It was a "catch 22" in which no positive outcome could be foreseen. He chose to deal with the negative energy world which was too absurdly irrational to be tolerated by any physicist worth beans, and Paul Dirac was one of the most rational creative geniuses of his time.

He wrestled with negative energies through all of 1929, trying to see if there was some way to keep the Dirac equation but get rid of the negative energy states.

Finally he submitted to his equations. His solution was to accept the negative energy states filling up the vacuum with a sea of negative energy electrons. He "solved" it by stating, as follows:

> "It is a bottomless sea, but we do not have to worry about that...We just have to think about the situation near the surface, and there we have some electrons lying above the sea that cannot fall into it because there is no room for them."

Thus the existence of the "real world" is the result of energy that comes out of an underlying "unreal world". It cannot fall back into the "unreal world" because there is no room left for it. Therefore we don't have to worry ourselves about the existence of the unreal world, as long as the real world can't disappear into it, according to Dirac!

If your point of view is metaphysical, then the above statement is both brilliant and incredible. Dirac fell prey to the solution of the fragmented pendulum. By extending its swing to the upper half, with a little metaphysical imagination, it may have been possible to accept the equations which posit the existence of negative energy as a real dimension even though it may be invisible and unmeasurable. Instead he dismissed it. That is the worst hole in quantum physics.

In the quontic psychological point of view, the discovery of negative energy states infers the inevitable existence of an invisible energy that underlies and transcends visible energy/mass. It's about the totality of the structure of the universe. It means that the real world can indeed disappear into the unseen world, and that the real world can manifest itself from the unseen world. It may also mean that Lorentz's equation and its conclusion that the speed of an electron may exceed the speed of light may also be correct. If this is so, it might turn out that the "invisible world", the Dirac sea, in which real particles exist and out of which they manifest, might even become tangible and real in some way at speeds faster than light-speed. The unseen universe with laws of its own, not defined by conventional physics and everyday reality, might also make up over ninety percent of the total universe, the famous missing mass.

Dirac rejected the "abnormality" of infinite and negative energies even though the attempt to renormalize - which certainly revealed important new dynamic relationships in physics - didn't eliminate the original "aberration". It simply denied it temporarily while physics continued attempting to renormalize the situation. Nevertheless, being a part of existence, the "abnormality" revealed itself in another form.

A "Here", "There" and "Elsewhere" Reality

To say we have to ignore the ocean and just pay attention to the waves because all we are able to do is measure the motion of the waves on top of the ocean appears extraordinarily unempirical and irrational to me. It's as though, because we did not have the equipment to measure the depth of the ocean science actually rejected the major part of the oceanic universe for the sake of what could be measured on top.

It's like saying we have to reject thought and feelings because we can't measure them directly, which is what physics does in rejecting consciousness as scientfic or real data. All we can measure is sound waves made by words which are the product of thought and feelings. But they, the measurements, are not intrinsically the thing-in-itself, they are neither sounds, thoughts nor feelings. Nevertheless, measurements in psychological tests are statistically organized, validated and experimentally proven techniques of evaluating thoughts, feelings and words, none of which have substance in themselves. Thoughts, feelings and sounds arise out of "virtual thoughts, feelings and sounds" which are not present to measurement until a person or persons agree to do that.

Are unconscious processes giving rise to conscious feelings and thoughts a metaphor for virtual electrons and real electrons in quantum physics? The "real" world in physics is the product of what it can measure and what it can measure leads to a measurement which, for some, becomes all that exists so that measurements become the things in themselves. As a result, physicists are still looking for the missing 90 to 99 percent of the mass of the universe, searching for it in black holes, in massive solar neutrinos ejected from the sun, in the microwave background, believing they still haven't found it. It is clear to me that it is already represented in the "ocean of invisible energy" in Dirac's formulation of the solution to the quantization of relativity. But that is a solution which can't be measured as an objective thing so it is not perceived as a part of the real world and therefore is not considered to be a solution to anything. It's a theoretical curiosity which has some application in formulations in quantum electrodynamics, but doesn't meet the qualifications for reality, just as the concept of the unconscious fails to meet scientific qualifications of reality.

That is, not unless you can regard <u>reality as a variable outcome or product</u> of the things that you are measuring and of the measuring instruments themselves, as we suggested earlier. Thus, reality is not the thing in itself that makes up the real world. Reality is a resultant or variable, a constituted result of other "here", "there" and "elsewhere" things and thus an outcome of the consequences of the dynamics of their "here", "there" and "elsewhere" actions and interactions. And, as it turns out, measurements on which reality depends in science can only offer a limited number of variables in the total (infinite) number of possible variables determining an incidence of reality "here".

Physical measurements can only include a small part of the matter, energy, light, etc. in the universe because all measurments are limited to what is measurable on that equipment. The equipment in our version of reality includes the human being and his limitations. The Copenhagen interpretation is therefore at the same time accurate and insufficient, not because it doesn't allow speeds in excess of light but because it omits the "elsewhere" which is also the conscious activity of the human part of the equation, and the real, functional existence of the virtual reality of physics.

Matter is defined by instrumentation because scientists basically don't trust anything else. Dirac, like most scientists, takes the position that only what can be measured, mathematically formulated and fit within the procrustean bed of formalized physics need be accounted for in reality; nevertheless, the omnipresent negative energy states recommend themselves otherwise. These rejected equations demonstrate and prove in accepted scientific terms that the detection screen provided through conventional physical experimentation does not include all that exists. It proves that a form of energy beyond the scope of current experimental research and its equipment does in fact exist and that we must continue to search for ways to bridge the gap between the seen and the unseen universe because they are both contributing to the variables of everyday reality.

Even behavioristic psychology, which attempted to determine human behavior through the maze running habits of mice and the pecking behavior of pigeons to make itself scientific, finally acceded that there is an invisible, unconscious world which must be included to understand 'rational' behavior. When will physicists give up their pecking stands?

Experimentation in cosmic rays, later, in 1932, revealed the existence of positrons, (virtual energy, antimatter, positive electrons) and from an embarrassment the negative energy states became a triumph for quantum electrodynamics and Dirac who won the Nobel prize for it in 1933. Essentially, though not admittedly, the prize was for the discovery that a good deal of the universe could not be seen because it existed in an infinitely negative state beyond zero point energy.

Transformation in Psyche and Atom

At the risk of being too obvious, it seems clear to me that our search for "impossible" concepts in physics that could relate to meta-physics was rewarded. Negative energy beyond zero point could not be measured because it did not appear to exist in a material form until antimatter, a positive electron, was discovered to represent the negative energy state. Is it too much to point out that the immaterial to the material state is exactly the kind of transformation we have been experiencing in psychic healing, in channelling, and past lives, to name just a few remarkable and puzzling energy transformations that have been exhaustively explored and reported in paranormal journals?

Physics always plays on the edges of known reality. For example, a recent report in Nature involving particle research by Drs. Aharanov and Casher at Tel-Aviv University examined the question of whether neutrons, which are particles which have no charge, and electrons, which have a negative charge, can interact. To everyone's amazement, it appears that a neutron can sense an electron from a distance without being evidently capable of experiencing a force generated by the particle's electric or magnetic field. Thus, although the neutron does not have an apparent electrical stimulus-response capability it somehow communicates with an electron which does have it, even at a distance. What is the mechanism by which the interaction takes place?

In 1959, Aharonov and Bohm discovered that even when a magnet is covered by a shield to prevent the transmission of a force to another magnet nearby, the phase of the electron wave function was altered, changing the shape of the wave in the receiving magnet.

> "Aharanov and Bohm predicted that this effect was due to a physical entity more fundamental than electric and magnetic fields: a potential, whose rate of change over space and time yields the electric and magnetic fields. After three decades, the Aharonov-Bohm effect has been demonstrated conclusively in experiments done on electrons traveling through a vacuum, and...in very small conducting wires at low temperatures." (Imry & Webb, 1989 [8])

Bohm and Aharonov propose that interactions of that type are possible because an electron creates "a potential field" (not unlike the "Dirac ocean") out of which actual electric and magnetic fields can emerge. The potential field is what may affect the neutron in the Ahranov-Casher experiment.

Additional, fascinating characteristics of the potential field is that it appears capable of conveying signals through "spooky action at a distance", as Einstein called it. In this case a positive electric charge will change its direction of movement without having to touch a negative charge, in which case no evident charges have been exchanged between particles. The effect implies that potentials - not actual fields, as had been thought - are what act directly upon charges.

Again, action in the real world is an emergent of energies that are not in themselves easy to identify on the physical level. This explanation, I would point out, is actually a description of the pilot-field of holographic theory.

But, it must be asked, without electric charge of its own, how can the neutron sense the presence of the potential field? The neutron, it is proposed, has a magnetic strength, called "magnetic moment", acting in a particular direction. The neutron's magnetic moment is what interacts with the electron's potential field. This theory was examined through experimentation recently and the ability of the neutron to respond to an elusive amount of energy in the electron's magnetic field was confirmed, as was said earlier.(Ruthen 1989[9])

The astounding thing about this experiment is that a theoretical potential energy in a non-existent field is being credited with positively affecting an unmeasurable magnetic strength in the electromagnetically neutral neutron! Furthermore, this work on the non-existent and hypothetical magnetic strength was confirmed by an experiment that actually measured the action of these energies only known by their effects upon each other since they do not follow the standard laws of physical operations. However, despite their inability to reject the experimental effects shown by means of the Aharonov-Bohm effect which depend upon non-existent, not palpable, physical energies, physicists will not accept the comparable self-evident results of psychic research.

Feynman, during his Nobel Prize award address in 1965 was somewhat more open to the acceptance of the implausible results that physics continually struggled against. At one point he stated:

> "In the face of the lack of direct mathematical demonstration, one must be careful and thorough to make sure of the point, and one should make a perpetual attempt to demonstrate as much of the formula as possible. Nevertheless, a

<u>very great deal more truth can become known
than can be proven</u>" (my underline) (P.453). And
later "...I believe there is no satisfactory quantum electrodynamics...even one that doesn't agree
with nature.... I think that the renormalization
theory is simply a way to sweep the difficulties of
the divergences of electrodynamics under the
rug. I am, of course, not sure of that." (Feynman
1985 P.454[10])

Renormalization is the attempt to discard parts of mathematical formulae that necessarily include infinities and zero
point energies, which are called divergences. "I am, of course,
not sure of that" is, I suspect, Feynman's sensitivity about
being so assertive that he would offend his colleagues, and
not be considered a major player on their team.

Another Impossible Conclusion

Dirac and quantum electrodynamics had produced additional disturbing equations for physicists. The equations
predicted that just as a boat is rocked by its own wake, an
electron's field interacts with its own electron. The interaction ultimately results in an energy that is infinitely strong,
giving the equations an infinite energy result when it was
supposed to give a finite result, and this could not be. This
problem of a particle's interaction with it's own electromagnetic field is called "self-energy".

Among the eminent physicists whose rational pragmatism was threatened by the mathematics of infinite energy
were Heisenberg, Pauli, and Oppenheimer. For many years
they were compelled by its very inexplicableness to deal with
the problem of a particle interacting with itself in its own
electromagnetic field generating infinite amounts of "self-
energy".

There is a strong anthropomorphism in that name, which,
when looked at from a psychological point of view is impos-

sible to ignore. Are we not also composed of electrons and therefore subject to the effects of negative energy and self-energy, engaging in an interaction with our own energy fields? If the problem is transferred to the domain of the human being then it suggests that the universe is made up of an electromagnetic field which has not only visible pragmatic electromagnetic effects but invisible pragmatic electromagnetic effects. This again veers into metaphysics and quontic theory. Its an effect whose strength may come from a universally infinite energy, a feedback effect from a universal energy field to its own visible energetic object. Essentially, this is what was discussed in the Bohm-Ahronov Effect. The display terminal for the feedback effect of self-energy could certainly be the consciousness capability of the human organism that enters into an energy realm which we have called fifth-dimensional.

The self-energy problem in physics may also represent a metaphor for the generation of energy between self and others. As a person acts upon his environment in three dimensional field relationships he also generates energy feedback within the environment which in turn energizes him, so that there is a continual feedback effect from a person's energy. Whatever kind of energy you infuse into your electromagnetic field must include persons within that field, and "as you sow so shall you reap" from the kind of energy that will be played back to you from the field. In this way you also create your own environment and have responsibility for whatever effects come from the energies which are the result of your own behavior. Thus, the dynamics of self-healing and illness of any kind, as well as relationships, may be generated by an invisible, infinite, but real self-energy field.

Energies are also being generated by other people, animals, and lower forms of life which create fields of self-energy by their behavior. These self-energized fields emanating from different life forms must interact with one another, perhaps creating a new energy-field gestalt from the totality of interactions.

To expand this notion of self-energy interactions with feedback processes in the environment, the effect would be a network of energy and feedback systems, including that sent out and received by the planet Earth, determining what happens at any one moment. The "butterfly effect" of chaos theory - a butterfly flapping its wings in the Amazon might affect the weather in London - the widespread if not infinite effect that may result from interactions among diverse and far flung energy fields is one of the phenomena that the new science of chaos has recognized and attempts to include.

In the Dirac equation, self-energy interactions between the particle and its field occur to an extent that is infinite. In terms of irrational science concepts, we have already seen that it is easy enough to integrate this into the domain of spiritual and transpersonal, paranormal energy fields. A person's actions interacts with fields of the determinable seen universe, generating energy interactions which, in becoming infinite, must transcend the known universe of quantifiable energy. It must apparently ultimately engage the totality of energy in the universe, including an unseen universe, and affect relationships with infinite energy that we call spiritual. Understanding the process by which the interaction between material and unseen energy occurs is what irrational science is about.

More to Renormalize

Infinite self-energy as a physics problem was aided and abetted by another irrational aspect of the problem of electromagnetic mass.

When moving through a resistant medium (like walking through molasses) the body feels as if it has gained weight, though it actually isn't heavier. In the case of electrons, there is no medium, apparently, for them to move through, yet, even in a vacuum, a moving particle gains mass due to self-energy interactions with its electromagnetic field. Furthermore, if the energy charge of an electromagnetic field becomes infinitely large, then the particle's electromagnetic mass must also become infinite. We have already found that due to Einstein's mass-energy equivalence equation neither energy nor mass can change without affecting the size of the other. Nevertheless, the infinite charge of energy and mass were rejected out of hand. "Both conclusions are patently false", state Crease & Mann, reflecting pragmatic physics' tunnel vision (Crease & Mann P. 94).

Gribbon, in his presentation of the situation, looked at it more openly.

> "Unfortunately, the same quantum equations that yield infinite solutions in QED also tell us that the energy density of the vacuum is infinite, and renormalization [getting rid of the infinities by manipulating the mathematics of QED equations] has to be applied even to empty space. When the standard quantum equations are combined with those of general relativity to attempt a better description of reality, the situation is even worse—infinities still occur, but now they cannot even be renormalized. Clearly, we are barking up the wrong tree", he states (Gribbin 1984).

A simple example of what is both right and wrong with renormalization is given by H.M. Georgi (Davies 1989).

> "Suppose I need a used car and I go to the only used car dealer in town and find that every car, when I start the engine makes a horrible scraping noise and, after a minute or two, starts smoking and smelling awful and stops running. But the dealer tells me that there is one car which starts the same way, but if I gun the engine and

> pound on the dashboard the scraping sound goes
> away and the car runs beautifully. Well, I try it
> out and it works! Terrific! I don't even have a
> decision to make. So I buy the car and it's a great
> car, just what I need. But somehow I can never
> stop wondering about what causes the horrible
> scraping noise." (Davies 1989 [11])

The horrible scraping noise is the continual reintroduction
of infinity into mathematical equations despite temporarily
successful attempts to get rid of it through gunning the
engine and pounding the dashboard - also known as
renormalization.

An Impossible Summary

Getting rid of the infinities became "the fastest game in
town" during the 1930's, and it certainly continues. When
Oppenheimer, of nuclear bomb fame, tried to get rid of them
he came to the depressing conclusion that, in quantum field
theory, electrons interact with a vacuum, that is, with nothing at all (that is, filled with an infinity of unmeasureable
energy). Dirac, making matters worse, said that the predictable effect of the interaction between the electron and the
vacuum was to reduce the total charge of the particle to zero.
Without any charge, a particle doesn't exist. Particles that
do not exist, virtual energy, virtual mass, a sea of negative
energy (electrons with a positive sign) that can't be seen—
nevertheless have to be proposed surrounding real electrons
because they are necessary to explain what can be seen. The
inevitable mathematics makes negative energy the predomi-
nant ocean of energy in the universe while matter is the
occasional bit of flotsam and jetsam found bobbing about on
the surface - this was conceptually conceivable but unbeliev-
able to right-minded physicists.

These impossible conclusions were delicately called "divergences". Divergences had to be eliminated from nature,

however, so new equations were projected which would balance off the impossible conclusions. When you can do that to arrive at finite answers successfully you have "renormalized" a theory.

Here's what Gribbon says about "renormalization":

> "Starting from the Schrodinger equation, the cornerstone of quantum cookery, the correct mathematical treatment of the electron yields infinite mass, infinite energy, and infinite charge. There is no legal mathematical way to get rid of the infinities, but it is possible to get rid of them by cheating. We know what the mass of an electron is by direct experimental measurements, and we know that this is the answer that our theory ought to give us for the mass of the electron cloud ('virtual positrons' surrounding the electron in every nucleus of an atom). So the theorists remove the infinities from the equations, in effect dividing one infinity by another. Mathematically, if you divide infinity by infinity you could get any answer at all, and so they say that the answer must be the answer we want, the measured mass of the electron. This trick is called renormalization."

In the chapters of this book I have been developing a paradigm to include in the normal what physics has attempted to renormalize, viz: the infinities, the less than zero energies, self-induced energy, plus as much as possible of what else we know that works in the quantum psychological domain. My goal is not to set paranormal psychology apart from the sciences but to show one way that we can incorporate both into a single paradigm, thereby broadening and unifying them. However, physics has to collaborate in this as well by looking again at their renormalized data to see whether it cannot indeed serve to consolidate the integration of the two, hopefully to arrive at the real Grand Unified Theory.

Dimensions of Time and Memory: Travelling the Q-Loop

The Fifth Dimension of Memory

The concept called "The Many Worlds Theory" in physics is fascinating because it borders on joining the metaphysical aspect of quontic psychology with its scientific aspect. Besides being one of the most famous scientific rejects it implies the strong probability of phenomena such as past lives. To bring many worlds into alignment with metaphysics and science, we should discuss time, space and memory in some depth. They are intimately related because if the many worlds theory is right, then we may live in multiple universes, ergo in past lives, simultaneouly with this one.

Whatever occurs in memory now must occur, for human memory to absorb and record it, in the three dimensional spacio-temporal dimension of contemporary events. Past life memory also happened in a three dimensional spacio-temporal framework and was contemporary for the person at the time that it occurred. How does it enter the "now" when it is no longer in the same framework as contemporary life memories?

Therefore there must be special laws for storage and recall of paranormal, and particularly past life memories. Some potential for special laws has already been described in the elaboration of quontic psychology. That potential will be continued here as well as in a discussion in another chapter about the speed of light and relativity. First let us specify some of the special characteristics of memory spacio-temporally in the familiar three dimensional framework.

What is familiar in what we remember depends heavily on the three dimensions that we know, to which we relate consciously. It may at first seem strange to see it pointed out that one of the external environmental factors affecting memory is dimensionality. That's because we have always taken three dimensional space for granted.

As a significant part of our physical experience, the spacial dimension in which we live both limits and vitally affects the characteristics of memory, as does our psychophysiological equipment which has evolved for survival purposes within three dimensions. This is so despite the scientifically recognized fact that time/space unifies into a fourth dimension, of which we have neither consciousness nor memory. What if other dimensions currently existed without our conscious participation in them? Wouldn't that revise our views about reality?

Giving it some thought, it will become apparent that whether we live in one dimension or in five dimensions will be a strong determinant of the kind of experiences we have, and therefore shapes a contribution to the form our memory will take. What characteristics are typical of dimensions?

A line is considered a one-dimensional space with very specific characteristics. If there were inhabitants on that line they could only move forward and back and would be totally flat. They would have to bump into each other and fight for the right of way, (like one-dimensional auto drivers who see the same parking space). They couldn't continue moving simultaneously without crashing because there are no possibilities of sideways, upward or downward movement. Such a person's memory would regard two dimensional space as something weird, a sci-fi fantasy at best, perhaps something to be longed for in his crowded one dimensional space, but nothing real.

A person living in a two dimensional space would be able to move sideways as well as forward and backward, getting out of people's way. He or she might be wide and long but as flat as one-dimensional man. Life and its memories would not even be as flexible as the memories of an ant which at least has something to look at in a third dimension. Three dimensions, the addition of height, would be the unheard-of impossible realm in a spatial expansion of mind which could never be a reality for the two dimensional person. He/she would be restricted to grand feats of imagination about three dimensions .

We accept three dimensional space without question because we live in it but our sensory-motor responses to three-dimensional space are something of a delusion in science as well as in mysticism. According to Einstein, three dimensional space does not exist independently of the dimension of time, and the laws of general relativity describe the symbiosis of space-time so they become relativized into four dimensions.

In relativity, the observer of an event is a participant in what is seen to happen because his position relative to a moving object determines the perceived time and place in which something occurs. (This will be developed in greater detail in later chapters.) In Special Relativity, the speed of light, which is a constant, becomes a determinant, along with gravity - without conscious effects on human functioning - in what happens to the mass and experience of objects accellerating in time. Gravity in turn affects light, but we are oblivious to gravity's effects even under average conditions. We are oblivious to the effects of relativity as well as to the entire realm of quantum physical existence even though both of these are fundamental to the existence and continuity of our universe. We would still be unaware of them if not for the invention of special instruments, beginning with the mind, then the telescope and microscope that have enlarged them into visibility in three dimensions. Life in three dimensional space is at least as limiting for us as two dimensional space would be for a two dimensional kind of being, and like him all we can do is fantasize about what life would be like in the next higher dimension.

It's strange to realize we actually live in a space determined by factors of which we have no conscious awareness.
We have no conscious memories of the fourth dimension any
more than we do of the Big Bang. Does that mean they don't
exist? Obviously not. There is a record that allows us to know
something of their history, as COBE has shown in recording
the microwave background which presumably began at the
Big Bang, but we exist consciously entirely in present time
and within its present parameters. This record of previous
history is everywhere in the rocks, oceans, organisms, stars
and universes beyond our own. In ways that science is just
now beginning to appreciate, it is also built into human
evolution and therefore into contemporary human functioning. This historical record, no matter in what form it appears,
is what I will be referring to as fifth dimensional memory.
In this way, it need not be restricted to three dimensional
form in human consciousness.

We see then that there are limits to our capacity to be
aware of dimensionality and therefore have no memories for
some dimensions and none for the quantum physical level of
existence, except for some persons as a concept. That limitation is relative to the capacities given to us by our physiological, sensory, intellectual equipment, which constitute
the physical product inherited within a particular environment. This gives us a clue that three dimensionality is a
construct that fits well with what our environment offers us
within a particular set of economically developed organismic
sensory-motor possibilities, in the interests of survival.

Within three dimensions we have developed a convenient
way to measure and organize our sensory work-a-day world.
Separation and boundaries between things, natural as well
as those we devise for our convenience, are established by use
of barriers and borders, which establish divisions. It then
becomes easier to quantify, organize, categorize and perform
other rational operations to gain mastery of our environment,
and of ourselves. Events occurring between conventionally
defined and accepted barriers and borders provide a reasonably logical form that help shape conscious memories within

our psycho-physiological organisms. Within the rationally developed structure of memories there is a built-in set of conventions that enables us to recognize them and to use them and reuse them automatically, facilitating the conduct of daily life.

Dreams are difficult because they often seem to elude or trespass beyond those conventions, and then we don't know how to use them. They require another level of understanding to interpret their meanings. Are they from the unconscious? Are they from another dimension of knowing? Is the unconscious another dimension or part of this one? Are dreams distorted memories or are they imaginative fictions? If not, what?

In the natural fifth dimensional universe, states with barriers may not exist at all. Why can't there be a memory that is "beyond memory" so to speak, that exists in a state whose boundaries are not defined by the first to third dimensions and by conventional audio-visual cues? Freud's proposition of the unconscious mind was such a concept in a way. It established the presence of a mental state whose dynamics were not the simple result of conscious everyday cues that fed rational ongoing remembering and forgetting. Nevertheless, its evidence became so strong that the unconscious mind became incorporated into psychotherapy first and now is easily generally understood to influence everyday affairs. However, it's boundary with consciousness is considered very leaky, and it's not scientifically acceptable. The boundary of phenomenological, unifunctional experience cannot be defined by science and by experimentation as it exists today.

Even within science, the boundary situation is ill-defined in the relationship between classical and quantum physics, as well as between many other fields of scientific study. For all practical purposes, physicists do not bother to differentiate the boundaries and borders between quantum and classical physics, although quantum mechanics as a whole describes a realm of subatomic reactions which classical physics cannot share.

Speculating on this question of the boundary between classical and quantum physics, J.S. Bell, writes,

> "A possibility is that we find exactly where the boundary lies. More plausible to me is that we will find that there is no boundary....On the other hand, it is easy to imagine that the classical domain could be extended to cover the whole. The wave functions would prove to be a provisional or incomplete description of the quantum-mechanical part....It is this possibility, of a homogeneous account of the world, which is for me the chief motivation of the study of the so-called 'hidden variable' possibility." [1] (P.30)

The above is Bell's way of stating that reality is unifunctional, after all.

What has this to do with memory? In Quontic Psychology I have proposed two basic dimensions of memory - the 3rd and 5th - which interact with each other. They are separated by different modes of functioning which creates differences and allows interactions. The search for "the hidden variable possibility", and the elusiveness of boundary conditions, implies that the barrier between the third and fifth dimensions also is an artificial construct created out of human perceptual and cognitive limitations. They are actually on an invisible continuum permitting a change in form and in modes of functioning via the quontic loop, allowing energies to be transformed during exchanges between them.

At present, physics has established strict barriers between itself and paranormal research e.g. between the third and the fifth dimensions. We have begun to examine the truth of that barrier and have found, and will continue to find, that it is full of holes. It's like the Berlin wall, ergo, someone built it and someone can tear it down. We are in accord with Bell's goal to develop a homogeneous account of the world. Later in this chapter we will explore the dynamics of the relationship between energy states such as memories in the third and fifth dimensions and speculate on how energy transformations occur through the principle of the action potential.

Practical and Impractical Time/Memories

It is clear that memories are not simply what we learn in school for exams or what we learn from our parents about behavior. They are implicit, if not explicit in every area of our physical as well as our psychologically deep functioning. Networks of organic, mnemonic, psychophysical relationships are what keep us functioning adequately in the everyday world, maintaining our assurance of survival, ability to work and grow and relate to others. However, this functional view of memory doesn't satisfy us when we attempt to search beyond the everyday level into paranormal, past life and even future life experiences.

Inevitably, when we look at memory on the practical level we place it in a three dimensional space and time frame. This means causal relationships between events determine our understanding of what's going on. Once you depart from the conventional way of thinking, the causal time frame gets shaken, and it no longer can explain events occurring beyond its limited parameters. In dreams and in paranormal experiences time may lose its causal connections. By better understanding what the causal time frame is like, we can understand the atemporal frame better.

Time in its essence is not an independent thing or object. Things that tell time, like clocks, or things we use for measurements, like meters, have no temporal qualities in themselves. They have moving parts and numbers whose fragmented relationship we can note and relate to within a technological structure that we use which we call measuring time. This relationship to measurement and the ability to control its stopping and starting on measurement devices is what is very basic to scientific experimentation.

When you stop the clock you don't stop time, you simply stop a mechanical counter. The movement of the counter or clock which we call time has become a variable that helps us to make judgements about other variables like speed of movement which is important for measuring changes in activities. However, time's material existence is not even as tangible as air or electricity which, though also unseen, create forces and resistances whose effects can be measured. Electricity has effects on objects which can be easily seen with the naked eye. Time doesn't have such a tangible, material effect.

Or does it? What about aging, rusting, deterioration of objects? Actually, they are the effects of ongoing natural biochemical, organic processes which are not caused by time but take place at a steady rate of change in accordance with the entelechy, the natural degradation of elements, sustaining the process. It's this steady rate and direction of change that we gauge with mechanical measuring devices and numbers and call it time.

For us then, time is a device we have created to measure movements and changes that take place in space. Timing this action, we call the movement speed, and acceleration. Movement may be very unpredictable and result in uncertain speed, as in a race, or it may be very regular and predictable as the length of a day and the rotation of the earth around the sun. In either case the mechanism we have created to measure time is predictable, if it's a timepiece that works well. We therefore have gained an orderly way of organizing our information. In its simplest calendar form, time is a measure of the length of lapses or distance between events in terms of the rotation of the earth around the sun, on a scale of seconds to years.

However, on any scale, large or small, time is a dependent variable because the measurement of it cannot exist without the presence of other factors such as space and measuring devices. Time can only be measured by us in the context of three dimensional space because then there is something that happens to an object by which we can measure changes, making the change "objective". There are then five interrelated factors on which time must depend for its measurability. These five factors will help us to define the contextual or structural aspect of memories, giving form to their contents.

Five Factors On Which Time Depends For Its Measurability:

1. Changes.

These may or may not be visible and have observable effects on material things. Aging is a change whose minute effects are not visible but whose long range effect is. The atoms in objects are always moving about but most of us will never see this because we don't use the equipment needed to make such microscopic phenomena visible unless we do research. We don't see the changes in temperature taking place in the molecules of water that we heat up for tea until the water boils.

2. Movement.

It's easy to see physical changes in spatial positions due to the movement of an auto, a bird or an airplane. This is what we most often measure with our timing devices. Most scientific experiments have relied on a time frame to measure physical change as a criterion by which to judge the outcome of the experiment. In Behaviorist psychology the rates of speed by which rats and pidgeons went through mazes or solved other obstacle problems was considered a criterion for learning capability. The same is true in I.Q, tests which presume to measure intelligence based on the correctness and speed of completing a task. Qualities such as insight, awareness, intuition are not given value on such tests because they can't be measured with a time factor so consciousness was rejected as a human function by behavioristic psychology, as it is today in science generally. These factors lack "objectivity". Time measurements require movement of an object in space, or a beginning and end of a defined action.

3. Physical Space.

Anything that exists in the material dimension has to exist in space. Without space there is no ability to perceive the movement of an object, whether the pattern from a diffraction grating made by a photon, the light bulb that lights up or goes out, something that rusts, the consequences on the face of the person who ages or the measurement of energy from colliding electrons in a super-collider. There has to be an "out there" in which we gauge the changes that take place in time's numerology. You cannot gauge the changes of an object in time without an awareness of its position in a spacial dimension. Of course, these first three items on which time depends for its measureability are intimately related.

4. Psychological Space-time.

A thought, a feeling, an impulse, an awareness, are events that take place in psychological space over a specific time. A mental event goes through a process of psychological and neurological refinement and alteration until it is either repressed or expressed. We are usually not even aware that this process is going on, but neurologists have been able to measure the miniscule amounts of time that impulses take to travel through the nervous system. All we may consciously be aware of is that we think, feel, or have an impulse to do something. If we do it, the outcome expressed in actions, words, music or pictures has a psychological effect on a perceiver. We become aware of a beginning and an ending to something being expressed and can estimate the time it took to do it.

Thought, feelings, and impulses, however, take up psychological space and time, prior to material physical space and time. Psychological space-time may or may not be expressed in behavior through which it can be measured.

Books take up psychological space-time, much more than they do physical space. It may take ten hours to read a book that took four years to write which covers fifty years of social change. A film may take two hours to depict several years, even decades, of a person's or a generation's life. We recount events in several minutes that may have taken several hours to happen.

We are able to distinguish between psychological and physical space-time. When we recall an event we understand the difference between its actual time span and the amount of time it takes us to tell it. When a person recalls a past life he understands the difference between the psychological space of that time period and the contemporary recounting time period. We depend a great deal on psychological space-time to record and report mental events that are correlated to events in physical space-time.

5. *Cognition of the Perceiver.*

Although the object measured in an experiment is "out there" the one who knows that time has passed is the perceiver, whether one or more persons. In recounting an event that took place in the past, whether in this life or a past life, the only person who has a knowledge of the time frame of the event is the person who experienced it. Communication is the process of a perceiver trying to give to others the same knowledge that one has oneself, to communicate the perceptions and the cognitions one has gained in the course of perceiving events. Though cognition, like feelings, may be subject to evaluation it too is a product of psychological space-time and not measureable in a time-space framework until it results in some form of behavioral expression.

If we put all of the above together and subsume them under a generic term, that term would not be beauty or truth or emotion, though they might arouse those kinds of sensations, but they could neatly subscribe to the function we have of ordering events in what we call "memory". Can you imagine the occurrance of an event that you remember without being able to put it into some kind of movement or change process taking place in space in a time duration, filled with yourself or another person as the perceiver? It is this process that gives human and other organisms a memory in a time/space frame or structure for events that have occurred in three dimensions.

The fifth dimension has rules of its own which transcend those of the third and fourth dimensions, transcending relativity as well as those of ordinary human functions.

Short, Long and Unlinear Memories

Ordinary memories, whether short term or long term, are about events developed in linear time in daily life in three dimensions using the recording facility of consciousness. Such memories, recorded as linear events in the past of this life, return in the present time and space of the perceiver generally influenced to some degree by present space-time. The converse is also true, namely, that events in the present may be influenced in the way they are perceived and remembered by events of the past.

If you question the reality of a memory you can call it imagination, or hallucination or a dream or some such, depending on how far from experienced reality the mental event seems to be. A memory is called real because it is based on remembered events known to have occurred within the linear framework. Something from imagination is not considered real because it does not come entirely from recognizable three dimensional, linear experience.

Then what is imagination and where does it come from? Like memory, imagination usually has the same five point framework — space/time movement, change, a perceiver, and cognition — that was a precondition for a causal memory. Therefore in terms of our definition, though imagination has a "time" dimension, just like memory, it is not necessarily represented in pure linear terms. The time frame is often jumbled, it isn't clear, so we don't ascribe a familiar space/time frame of real events to imagination. Familiar structures and sequences are often lacking, times and places and real forms can become jumbled up and confusing, so without the linear spacial framework we don't consider it real. Because it is lacking a set of remembered three dimensional events in linear relationship to each other, imagination has a product which isn't familiar to consciousness as a linear past recall is. Familiarity due to its linear components appears to be an additional characteristic that we require of recall before calling it a memory.

Strange to say, past life memory can be distinguished from imagination because it has the same linear components that a present life memory does. It has a framework in its own space and time that is progressive, is orderly and logical in the way events are recalled. Feelings are experienced and thoughts can be expressed in comprehensible ways in the here and now during past life regression. It does not fit the bill for imagination.

Imagination

Where does imagination come from?

The question implies that the boundary between imagination and realistic memory is rigid, consequently, people ask whether a past life experience is due to imagination or due to memory, too. Imagination, dreams, illusions and hallucinations lack a clear linear reference point in daily life; they manifest looser boundaries in regard to reality. Nevertheless, they must have components that refer to three dimensional types of events in time and space or they couldn't be referred to at all. They are organically the product of the same process as real memory is, however they are less subject to the linear level and therefore less likely to have a behavioral reference in familiar time and space.

I am suggesting, much as Freud describes dreams, that imagination is made up of structures which are a compromise between total repression of everything and the expression of unacceptable events, ideas and thoughts buried in the unconscious. They are thus difficult to understand, lacking a measureable time-space framework in their manifest form. This may come about because the hallucinating person himself, for instance, is unable, due to traumatic growth experiences, to separate and identify past and present, actual from distorted linear content. By the same token, whether it drives the patient into intense fear, rage or whatever, it is also a legitimate expression of that person's relation to his experience in the present moment and deserves respect as such instead of judgement and condemnation as insanity.

It is often the same stuff out of which dreams and the creative arts, whether drama, painting or dance are made. The difference is in the structure given the latter within the linear, relevant framework of present space-time. Freud gave us the first clues to this process, which are simply elaborated and placed in another perspective here.

The sources of an hallucination are likely to reside in terrifying events that could have occurred in early childhood in this life, or in a past life. As in dreams, the content has been disguised in an attempt to repress the source of the terrifying feelings. However, powerful emotions are not that easily disposed of and they create a way to become expressed by building a structure, like a scaffolding, more or less linear, on which to hang the repressed emotional events. The creative, distorting, disguising work of dreams, hallucinations and the imagination can make their linear references unrecognizable. The outcome is what we call imagination, or a creative work of art, or a fictional story or an hallucination, or a dream, depending on the scaffolding and materials available in present space-time to the person. Therefore, imaginative work of any kind may be regarded as a symbolic, metaphorical statement that represents a coalesced internal psychophysiological state whose sources in memory may be disguised for the sake of representing a presently motivated energy or drive - such as to express and heal a disturbing problem. It's urgency is often due to the survival - homeostatic axis on which it turns.

Past life memories in particular, for the most part, express this axis of homeostatic, survival experiences and issues in their content. For this reason, in terms of its effectiveness for the purposes of psychotherapy, the question of the reality of a past life is irrelevant. The experience of it offers a fuller understanding of oneself and one's problems in the present linear frame. For the purposes of a scientific description of reality it is not provable, as yet.

Neither does that mean that a past life regression is not a memory of an event that occurred in reality. As stated earlier, it differs from imaginative productions in that it has a completely recognizable linear, rational, spacetime set of references. We will therefore explore the possibility of the reality of past lives by looking further into ideas that have come from science.

According to the Many Worlds Theory, there is even the possibility that we exist and have experiences that come from more than a single space-time framework simultaneously. That can be a frightening notion because the boundaries of linear space-time will be severely shattered if one accepts the Many Worlds Theory. That's why it has not found acceptance in the conventional physics community, even though nothing has ever been found wrong with it mathematically. Given its framework it apparently will never be experimentally proven by research in the form in which it stands today. Nevertheless, it is another valuable door, although coming from physics, to the fifth dimension.

Many Worlds — Many Times

Look, it cannot be seen - it is beyond form.
Listen, it cannot be heard - it is beyond sound.
Grasp, it cannot be held - it is intangible.
These three are indefinable;
Therefore they are joined in one.
From above it is not bright;
From below it is not dark;
An unbroken thread beyond description.
It returns to nothingness.
The form of the formless.
The image of the imageless.
It is called indefinable and beyond imagination.
Stand before it and there is no beginning.
Follow it and there is no end.
Stay with the ancient Tao,
Move with the present.
Knowing the ancient beginning is the essence of Tao.
— Lao Tse [1]

Cueing in on Time

Lao Tse is stating above that our three-dimensional experience of being in the world needs to give way to the aspect of experience that is intangible and unreal, in which there is no such thing as past, present and future. It is an experience beyond all sensory experience which itself is fragmented until it is given up which only then allows us to experience the unity underneath and beyond everything.

In experiencing the Tao you will know all that there is to know, including "the ancient beginning" of all experience which is neither beginning nor end, only "the unbroken thread" of formless, imageless existence. And the way into the essence of Tao is through the moving changes flowing in the present.

In the pragmatic Western mode, I like to relate to time in terms of a billiard table on which are set three balls — past, present and future. Imagine that they are in such a relationship that, due to electromagnetic forces, hitting one with the cue ball means that you have to hit the other two. They are arranged on the billiard table, our electromagnetic field, in such a way that hitting one angles off to hit another ball which angles off to hit the third each time, no matter which one you hit first. They continually attract each other and collide due to the electromagnetic forces between them.

We are the players in this billiard game. We may think we are able to direct the cue ball only to the present, but inevitably we find we also have hit the past and the future, or think we are hitting the past and find we are hitting the present and the future as well; or we think we are only planning the future but we are affecting the present, as well as drawing on our history in the past - and changing the effects of that history itself. There is an invisible tie that binds all present actions into a network beyond the appreciation of our everyday sensory and perceptual capabilities.

Concerning the Origin of Time and the Universe

There exists another kind of related problem in three dimensional time and space for physicists. They are concerned about the reason for the direction of time, trying to find out what happened to make the past become the past instead of remaining the present; in other words, why time started taking a direction at all. The direction, according to the law of entropy is toward dissolution of energy, in keeping with the expansion of the universe. Entropy is like a dye which will dissolve in water, gradually coloring the water uniformly. In terms of the universe this means that the energy in the universe may run itself down through continual expansion until it disappears into nothingness.(Prigogine 1984 [2]) At that point all boundaries and fragmentations which have constituted three dimensional life experience will become dissipated. In the scientific method, loss of all boundaries means the extinction of living matter. In mystic ideas, loss of boundaries means returning to an original source and its limitless state of being. The present thinking about the dissolution of the universe through expansion is not definite. There are two other scenarios: one, that the universe might contract into itself and become a black hole and another that it might just continue to expand, slowly and indefinitely. No one scenario is certain and all are possible.

Memory, like time's arrow and the beginning of the universe, with its innumerable challenging questions defies a reasonable psychophysiological, or metaphysical explanation. Where and what is the unconscious before it becomes conscious? There is no known locus in the brain for unconscious memories though there appear to be brain parts that function to retrieve and to store short term and long term memories. Until memories are called into action for any reason, they remain in an undifferentiated unconscious state. How and where? The best we can physiologically say is that the brain's neurones fire in a patterned fashion when stimulated by receptor nerves. Patterns of neurochemical receptors somehow store impulses in the nervous system which are what are retrieved, in our understanding of the psychophysiological aspect of memories. Out of the stuff of memory we create and sometimes fictionalize what we want to know to make ourselves feel more comfortable and secure in our lives. Thus we create and recreate everything from our self-concept to our social institutions and perhaps our revered sciences as well. In the self-concept, memory may become a creative act. Just so, in science, knowledge may become a creative act. Thomsen states:

> "The historians did not experience the past. Likewise the crime detective, who 'knows' the quantum mechanical formula intuitively, constructs a variety of scenarios and evaluates the probability that they predict what will be found. So in science also, we make a cosmology from the data probability has given us." (Thomsen. P. 347)

The personal history we create, the cosmology we deduce—do they start with memories that are based in real events, or are they concoctions of our creative unconscious using possibility as the baseline for probability, going from there to the presumption of "knowledge" and "ultimate truth" and "science"?

Later in this chapter we will discuss light cones, a concept of Stephan Hawking's, which provides a continually expanding energy model for the universe based on the expansion of time. However, Hawking has introduced a twist into expansion in showing how light cones could expand equally into the past as well as into the future.

The issue of time's direction, or time's arrow, was large enough for it to be one of the concerns of a meeting of physicists held at the Fermi National Accelerator Laboratory in Batavia, Ill. called the Workshop on Quantum Cosmology. This meeting was reported by D.E. Thomsen for Science News in June of 1987 in which he stated:

> "If we trace the expansion of the universe backwards we eventually come to a point in history when the universe was so small that it had to behave as a whole as a quantum mechanical system. Figuring out how the present came out of the past is the problem." (Thomsen 1987 [3])

That simple question involves incredibly complex dynamics which may never be fully unravelled. How the present came out of the past means how an infinitesimal bit of energy (in physical size though incredibly massive in energy size) exploded via "the Big Bang" into the world as it is today. Much information has apparently accumulated about the earliest micro-seconds, but not about the explosion itself. Now, however, at the beginning of the 90's other theories have made their appearance which question the big bang's validity.

Aside from the question of the physics of material functioning in relation to the direction of time, there must be some way to understand the psychological relationship of living organisms to time. Their relationship to time is complicated by the facts of life cycles, memories, sensory-motor capacities and consciousness that somehow evolved out of the same process as the rest of the physical universe. Physics does not concern itself about such matters however, and other sciences such as archeology, psychology and paleontology attempt to find answers to those less definable, less measurable questions.

Beyond the Big Bang

The Fermilab meeting had to do with the "ground state" of the universe, or the simplest possible conditions under which it could function. Our question is the meta-physical one: whether there could have been a point of zero diameter and therefore infinite space, zero time and therefore timelessness, no laws and therefore inherently all laws existing simultaneously synchronistically, prior to and supporting the Big Bang. How can we encompass such a possibility in our known reality - nothing and everything seem to be such extreme opposites - (taking further poetic license) unless they exist on a transcendental Moebius curve in whose flow they merge.

An essential ingredient in recognizing the flow of time is the process of change, whether in the flow of seasons, aging, entropy, destructive forces or reconstruction. Insofar as these are recognizable and measureable in terms of hard data which subscribe to the scientific method, it is possible to pinpoint measurements in time. In the science of physics experientially recognizable processes which are not measureable through time as hard data are not acceptable as valid. Therefore, without finding an answer to the question of the first millisecond of the universe the arrow of time cannot be adequately described so the origins of time's direction remains an unknown. The origins of the universe inevitably remains pertinent, however, to the meta-physical question of a dimension of existence without hard data. Again, as we have done throughout this book, we can see if there are ideas in physics which overlap those of meta-physics and/or psychological states of being to determine whether there may indeed be a relationship between physical and meta-physical data.

The Plasma Theory

Recently, another theory about the origins of the universe has developed to compete with the big bang theory. It is more compatible with our notion that time is only an artifact of civilization, and is not intrinsic to the formation of the universe. It states that "the universe may have evolved out of a vast sea of plasma", according to A. L. Peratt in The Sciences. As an alternative to the big bang theory, the plasma theory is finding support because it offers solutions to problems that the big bang has left unanswered or answered with inaccuracies when compared to the data.

A plasma is a state of free electrons, (negative charge) existing everywhere in the universe which is a good conductor of electricity. When its negative charge interacts with positive charges built up along the ground the interaction creates a channel of discharge manifested as lightning. The description of plasma uses such phrases as "plasmas are dominated by electromagnetic forces and fields", or plasma forms "multiple strands of conducting current", and "Experiments conducted in 1952 indicated that if the magnetic field-aligned current of a plasma is bent into a closed loop, the plasma takes the shape of a torus, or doughnut".

To continue with the description of plasma in physics, Peratt says,

> "...In recent decades investigators employing a wide array of sophisticated devices, including radio, ultraviolet and high-energy telescopes, particle counters and magnetic field probes, have shown that the cosmos is teeming with electrically charged sub-atomic particles. It is now estimated that 99.999 percent of the observable matter in the universe is made up of plasmas....Thirty years of space research has revealed the solar system to be a veritable sea of plasma, invisible to optical telescopes yet traversed by complex, interacting electric and magnetic fields....The computer simulations, supported by recent observations of intergalactic plasmas, give strong evidence that plasmas do indeed play a primary role in the formation of the cosmos.

> "...Like predawn mist beading on a spiderweb, the observable cosmos condenses out of the plasma background in progressively smaller steps, eventually forming stars, planets and moons. There is no expansion, and there need not be any final crunch. Unlike the universe envisioned in the big bang model, the plasma universe evolves without beginning and without end: it is indefinitely ancient and has an indefininte lifetime in store."

Is Peratt a Taoist? Is it a coincidence that he describes a "universe [that] evolves without beginning and without end; it is indefinitely ancient and has an indefinite lifetime in store". Or is it that Lao Tse's intuition is slowly becoming confirmed by scientists who are restricted to using the scientific method? The gap, if one accepts the valid existence of both forms of knowledge, is slowly closing between metaphysics and empirical physics.

The plasma concept is also unmistakably similar to the quantum theories of virtual photons and electrons, which announced the existence of virtual energy, mass and light. It sounds like still another version of Dirac's invisible, infinite sea of electrons, the blooming, buzzing confusion around a visible electron out of which the tendency for something has transformed itself into the tangibility of something.

The plasma concept for the background energy behind the cosmos makes it easier to say that the universe began with wholeness, which is simplicity itself, because then it is total fluidity of interacting components, or a state of no components, without boundaries. How did this state of simplicity, of total balance—total chaos if viewed from the 3-4D perspective—in the past, change? Was the simple state of plasma a precursor from which the Big Bang erupted, and might time and further experimentation reveal that the plasma theory has validity without a Big Bang, as Peratt suggests? And if, as Von Neumann states, consciousness is the necessary factor in the transition from wave to particle, and that transition could have been started with the Big Bang - could consciousness also have been a factor in the transformation from a simple state of plasma wholeness into formation of the material universe?

We don't actually know how the universe began. Given simplistic origins, you can start with a matrix of probabilities for the origins of the universe, says Thomsen (1987). You set up a number of possibilities and see which is the most probable. Ultimately, he says, the most probable is the one you probably remember.

"...Bring it down to us and our measurements, and then to the probability that we will have certain data in our memories. Here the theory becomes very much an information theory...that history is what you remember...and what is in our memory banks depends on probability".

In the end, Thomsen brings us back to the psychological factor and consciousness. The data in consciousness is the data determined by the joint possibilities of our histories and the probability of remembering certain aspects of that data. We know that here and now memory is selective, sometimes to the extent of creating delusional distortions, sometimes relatively reliable, probably never totally accurate. What is remembered in ordinary daily life often serves some special purpose - to pass an exam, to make ourselves look good, to get the better of someone in an argument, or to avoid the painful aspects of an experience by forgetting it and putting it out of memory. Therefore, all you can represent of the truth is what you remember. It's not even metaphysical, until you apply it to cosmology and the history of the universe. Then, as I've suggested before, memory is universal and homeo-static, serving survival of the cosmos as well as individual organisms.

On the scale of the cosmos and of the history of mankind, there would appear to be a "memory bank" of consciousness, the quontic warehouse, larger than our own with which individuals like Lao Tse and societies like the Tibetan Bud-dhists had better contact. In the West we are too imbedded in our empirical rationalism through which we delude our-selves into believing we can attain a pure scientifc objectivity to ever trust a "memory bank" or simple consciousness for knowledge, ignoring that our cognitive basis for knowledge is most often intuitive, subjective, and probabalistic. At least analogically one might say that memory is quantumized, that is, that it comes in packets of various sizes, that it's entry into consciousness depends on the dynamical inputs of the remembering person, and that what does come from memory banks into consciousness is not certainty but a selection of alternative possibilities.

Memory, whatever its origins or sources, enters into psychological experience. Basically, psychological experience is interwoven with the conventional three-dimensional rigidity of daily life and scientific method. What would it mean for us to release ourselves from the straitjacket of three-dimensional reality? What would a core memory of life, of the origins of the universe be like, if we could ever experience it?

Would it be something like the Buddhists have described, a state of non-being which is a state of total wholeness, a fifth dimensional state? Could the earliest separation out of the matrix of wholeness, of the birth of the universe from its womb into individuality, whether harmonious or chaotic, have been an event which was a transformation from an unboundaried to a boundaried state, from an unboundaried wave to a boundaried particle, from a virtual neutron which is neither positive nor negative to an electron which takes a charge to become manifest in three dimensional form?

There is some indication from current theories in physics that a bridge is needed into psychology, or worse, into metaphysics. Einstein acknowledged that relativity was only partly rational science. According to Hawking the quantum theory of gravity allows a space-time that has no boundaries, stating that "space-time would be like the surface of the earth only with more dimensions....The universe would just BE." Like plasma or even before the something of plasma and more like Lao-Tse's unimaginable universe? (P. 135-136). Isn't it that deep accessibility to an unconscious source, or to the quontic warehouse, that makes a genius like Einstein, or a Mozart or a Freud possible?

Perhaps, if the plasma theory is accurate, the familiar universe arose from a waveform of electromagnetic information that was formless - to give rise to a form and a boundary (like a lightning flash) which makes the information available to us in a three dimensional form whose experience we call memory, and sometimes intuition, and sometimes science when it has been formulated according to conventional rules. This notion fits very well with the idea that memory is evolutionary and cumulative, that it has evolved along with consciousness and returns in the unconscious to the origins of the universe, manifested in such records as Tibetan philosophy and the less tangible Akashic records, as well as in works of genius. (Eccles 1985 [4]) Genius finds a form to express a memory of the divine which intuitively we all recognize and accept.

In memory banks , there is a consciousness potential. Let us hypothesize that memory is an outcome of an interaction occurring when an unformed plasma takes a form. Consciousness in an unformed plasma state (the fifth dimension) becomes sensory by passing through some sort of barrier, going from nothingness into somethingness - passing the barrier, separating into form, time, and space from the uniformity of simple wholeness into three dimensional sensory, formed, material existence. Thus, also, a suggestion about turning wave into particle. Admittedly, images of a universe changing from nothing-formed into something-formed is almost as amorphous as going through a Black Hole (a something formed) into a universe with other dimensions.

I'll take poetic license into mellifluous metaphor by stating: A Black Hole—that's the eternal womb of the unborn universe becoming infinitesimally expanded.

Perhaps it all began when "The Whole of Consciousness" suddenly had a thought for the first time and it was so exciting that it set off an explosion that shook and changed the universe by creating differentiated consciousness - that was like the Big Bang - when the plasma struck cosmic lightning. We made the consciousness-explosion into metaphysical memory and then into science. We still grope on our hands and knees through memory and through science looking for answers. We weren't born too long ago.

What we have been discussing up to now in this chapter is, for the most part, the material of psychology, philosophy and poetry and something about what physicists have to say regarding space and time. It is not idle speculation but is leading us toward some additional concepts in quontic psychology.

Now let's become grounded again - that is, return to scientific theory -in order to take a further look at what some of the physicists, such as Stephan Hawking, think.

A Brief Encounter with Topology in Physics

Spacetime is the name given to the four coordinates of space plus time in relativity. Since our sensory equipment is only developed to handle three dimensions, we can't physically imagine four dimensions, but in physics fourdimensional spacetime is real. In Newtonian physics as in daily life, the arrow of time moves forward from the past into the future in three dimensions.

In quantum mechanics there is no distinction between past and future nor any need to distinguish between them. Time's arrow from past to present to future seems to be a strictly Newtonian three dimensional macrocosmic phenomenon. The concern we have in our daily lives about accessing the past or planning the future is also very connected to humanity's three dimensional consciousness, as we have already seen.

Past and future are directions in time's arrow which in physics involves the speed of light. It may seem fortituous to attempt to relate the factors of the speed of light in space and time to memory and consciousness, but an open mind is an advantage. It isn't as far-fetched as it seems at first glance, and Hawking leads the way. In what follows I am presenting Stephan Hawking's way of representing spacetime in his book A Brief History of Time[5]. His presentation is conceptual and toplogical. I will be expanding his conceptualization to include human memory and consciousness.

We have already seen that the circles made by a stone hitting the water that create an interference pattern are no different in their physical dynamics from light waves which cause interference patterns in the two-holed diffraction grating. However, instead of seeing waves of light as if they are spread out on a horizontal two-dimensional surface of water, imagine the waves spreading out vertically upward in a three dimensional field from the point of impact. In the topological diagram on the next page, Figure 17., *Space and Time a.*, the event in which the stone hit the water at point P in the present spreads out in ever-larger concentric circles into future spacetime.

The event of the stone hitting the water takes place in the present moment and each concentric circle marks a widening movement in seconds of time while its increasing diameter also marks its vertical growth in space. The resulting figure is a cone as shown in the lines in the time expanded concentric circles. The cone extends upward into the future from the point in the present when the stone hit the water. It will also extend backward into the past in a second cone going in the opposite direction in spacetime. (See Figure 18., *Space and Time b.*)

Many urgent questions affect my consciousness when I look at Hawking's topology of spacetime. What happens when there are many cones developing out of many stones hitting the water at infinitesimal intervals of spacetime interactions? Wouldn't that resulting multitude of cones be analogous to the incredible number of spacetime events occurring in a person's, a city's, a country's, the world's lifetime? What if each person's life is a series of continuous stones hitting the water (present moment in time) creating cones of spacetime going in both past and future directions continuously? When a multitudinous number of events create cones in spacetime, doesn't this also create interference patterns when the cone of one event intersects with the cone of another event in a person's life, or when the cone of one person's life intersects the cone of another person's life, and indeed when the cone of one society intersects the cone of another society? If they become interference patterns do

SPACE AND TIME

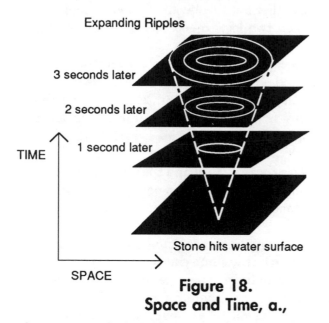

Expanding Ripples

3 seconds later

2 seconds later

1 second later

TIME

Stone hits water surface

SPACE

Figure 18.
Space and Time, a.,

the event in which the stone hit the wate in the present spreads out in ever-larger concentric circles into future spacetime.

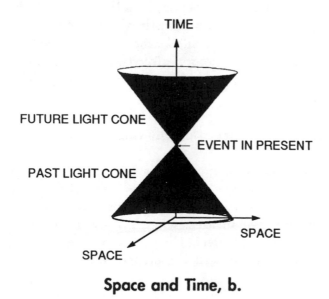

TIME

FUTURE LIGHT CONE

EVENT IN PRESENT

PAST LIGHT CONE

SPACE

SPACE

Space and Time, b.

they follow the usual rules for intersecting patterns, that is: two highs merge and create a greater high, a merging high and low wipe each other out to a levelled playing field? And what happens when two lows meet? (Suggests something very depressing).

Finally, since a cone is created from a spacetime which includes past as well as future time, what are the effects of past-past interactions, present-past interactions, present-future interactions and future-future interactions among cones? The complexity of possibilities begins to look overwhelming.

Unfortunately for the difficulty and the significance of our extension of his model, Hawking was not speculating when he described the topology of cones in spacetime. He stated,

> "...Maxwell's equations predicted that the speed of light should be the same whatever the speed of the source, and this has been confirmed by accurate measurements. It follows from this that if a pulse of light is emitted at a particular time at a particular point in space, then as time goes on it will spread out as a sphere of light whose size and position are independent of the speed of the source. After one millionth of a second the light will have spread out to form a sphere with a radius of 300 meters; after two millionths of a second, the radius will be 600 meters; and so on." (P.24,25).

Hawking then makes the following statement:

> "The situation, however, is quite different in the general theory of relativity [from the one in Newtonian theory]. Space and time are now dynamic quantities: when a body moves, or a force acts, it affects the curvature of space and time—and in turn the structure of space-time

affects the way in which bodies move and forces act. Space and time not only affect but also are affected by everything that happens in the universe." (P. 33)

It is repeatedly brought to my attention that frequently physicists, no matter how brilliant and enlightened, discuss events in physics as if they had no consequences for the human race. Fritjof Capra in the Tao of Physics made the first serious attempt to correct that, but his message, with a few exceptions such as those already noted, has not permeated the physics community. Humanity is an integral part of the notebook of events described in the networking of atoms, molecules, relativity and quantum mechanics. If light, in Hawking's model, forms a cone which expands its diameter at a ratio proportionate to the speed of light and can extend into the past as well as into the future simultaneously, thereby affecting everything in existence, then we have here a model for human energy existing simultaneously in past as well as future times into infinities past and future. If not, he has no right to make his last statement.

I will therefore assume that the cone model of space-time includes the human experience, unquestionably. If it is not true for the human experience then it is not true for the totality of physical experience. The consequences radiating from the cone model are as difficult as they are enormous, but they also appear to me to be obvious.

First, however, there's more to the topology of light cones in spacetime. Says Hawking,

"The past and the future light cones of an event P divide space-time into three regions. The absolute future of the event is the region inside the future light cone of P. It is the set of all events that can possibly be affected by what happens at P. Events outside the light cone of P cannot be reached by signals from P because nothing can travel faster than light." (See Figure 19., *Else-where*, on the next page.)

To which I'd add the observation that this restriction comes from the speed of light limitation and therefore may apply only within the relativistic framework in which it is described. The rules about the way the universe works have been fathomed only as far as relativity has taken us. Before Einstein, the rules went as far as Newton could take us, before that it was Kepler, Galileo, and so on. Some scientists periodically have the strange notion that all the rules have been discovered and there is nothing left but a little mopping up to get everything squared away.

Although supported substantially by many experiments coming out of relativity it is the belief of some physicists whose notions we have already examined that the limitation on the speed of light is itself a relative statement. Hawking makes a very circumscribed statement saying nothing can travel faster than light so that events outside the light cone cannot be reached. We don't actually know that - all we do know is that physicists at present do not have the means of sending, receiving, or determining whether there are signals outside the light cone.

In the case of light arriving on earth from distant parts of the universe, says Hawking:

> "...the light that we see from distant galaxies left them millions of years ago, and in the case of the most distant object that we have seen, the light left some eight thousand million years ago. Thus, when we look at the universe, we are seeing it as it was in the past [eight thousand million years ago]." (Hawking, P.28)

Of course it is a very different thing to see light coming from the past of a star as it was physically eight million years ago compared to looking down the history of a light cone whose

Space and Time

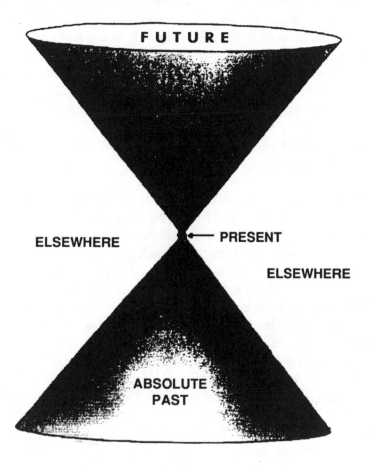

**Figure 19.
Elsewhere**

Events outside the light cone of P cannot be reached by signals from P because nothing can travel faster than light.

subject matter is the memory in consciousness telescoping into the past of a person's life to see how he lived eight hundred or even eighty years ago. The psychological instance is much more difficult to explain because it has no empirical equipment to examine it. The only equipment available to do that at present is consciousness. It is the most peculiar characteristic of the human being that he has access to a consciousness that can record and examine itself but does not subscribe to scientific methods of research.

Interactional Dynamics Between Time, Light and Consciousness

Can we perform the remarkable feat of entering physical light cones with past and future dimensions through a consciousness which also has past and future dimensions simultaneously? Is there a common denominator between consciousness and light cones which allows a common energy to intercourse between them? Perhaps there is. Light photons are energy bundles or quantumstuff made up out of electrons radiating electromagnetic energy waves outward. Electromagnetic radiation is measurable in terms of frequency of waves, wavelength, intensity, and wave amplitude, and in quantum mechanics by the laws of probability. Electromagnetic radiation is also a prime ingredient in the cellular and nervous network of the human organism where consciousness manifests itself most completely. It seems almost trite to point out that we are also a dependent variable, changing our perceptions, biochemistry and neurology as a result of the actions of light photons and electromagnetism present in the universe.

Since light is measured by frequencies and wavelengths, perhaps we may some day manipulate our electromagnetic functions, (experienced as thought and consciousness) as some say we could, to enter vibrational energies of photons, and therefore of light cones, which will enable us to transport ourselves, by means of consciousness, with the medium of light and of electromagnetic energy, through time and space. (It reminds me of the famous "Beam me up, Scotty" in Star Wars.) In that case, we would be entering light cones in their physical aspect through consciousness.

There are some intriguing consequences arising from this notion. Is this a metaphor expressed in topological terms or a real description of what happens when a past life is recalled and experienced?

It is quite useful as a topological metaphor. If we suppose that we know two persons whose past life light cones have intersected and overlapped we can probably diagram and mathematically quantify the amount of their past interactions. Taking a third person's past light cone and seeing how it interacts with the first two will provide the degrees of interaction these three persons may have had with each other. If we then project the light cones of these three people into the future, from point P present, perhaps adding a fourth person, we can predict how much future interaction these four people are likely to have. In the hands of a mathematician, this toplogical model could probably develop into several scientific looking formulae, if it could solve the chaotic element to estimate the chances that other unpredictable events will occur that will also affect the topological formula. (See Figure 20., *Three Cone Past Lives*, on the next page. Also see Figure 21., *Four Cone Future Lives*, a topological view of past life and future life interactions, arrived at by expanding Hawking's ideas.)

The Many Worlds Interpretation

Hawking's topology of spacetime leads us directly toward another past oriented explanatory concept in physics arising from the particle-wave dilemma. There is in physics a theory which is "irrational" proposed by Hugh Everett in a paper published in 1957, while a graduate student in physics at

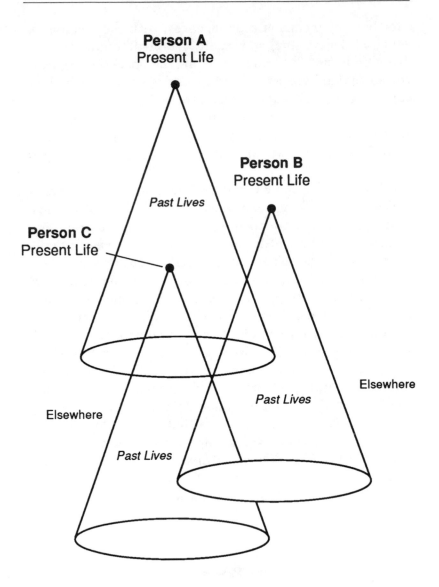

Person A
Present Life

Person B
Present Life

Past Lives

Person C
Present Life

Elsewhere

Past Lives

Elsewhere

Past Lives

Past Lives

Figure 20. Three Cone Past Lives

A topoligical view of past life interactions, arrived at by expanding Hawking's idea.

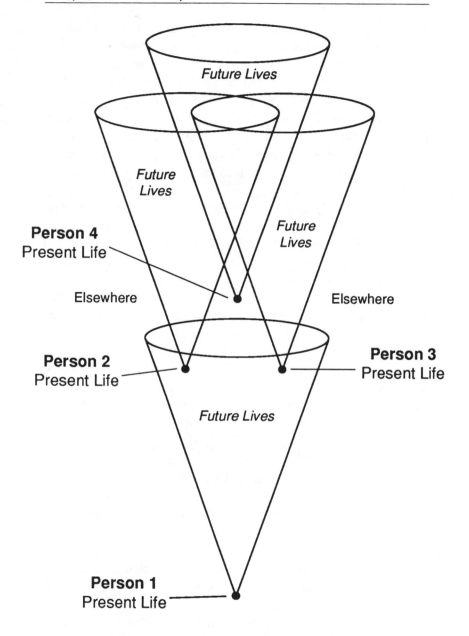

Figure 21. Four Cone Future Lives

A topoligical view of future life interactions, arrived at by expanding Hawking's idea.

Princeton, which enables us to use physics for an additional turn of the kaleidoscope, incorporating memory, perhaps unintentionally, into the structure of concepts described above. It was not intended to be a theory about memory, but it is nevertheless intricately related to the function of memory. It is called the "Many Worlds Interpretation", a quantum theory of cosmology which includes in its calculations the Copenhagen interpretation. It takes the single and double slit experiment that gave rise to the principle of indeterminacy discussed in the chapter on quantum physics a step further into an indeterminate number of possibilities. The fascinating thing about this outrageous theory, is that it too, like the Bell Theorem, and the past and future light cones of Hawking, is solidly grounded in the now accepted mathematical equations of quantum mechanics.

Taking the equations further, mathematicians have discovered that four-dimensional space can take many different topological routes, leading to very remarkable, different forms. "In the realm of four-dimensional exotic spaces, infinitely many ways exist to do calculus. Each exotic space has its own appropriate collection of expressions."(Peterson 1989 [6]) This observation was not developed to prove the many worlds idea, but it certainly can represent mathematical support for its scientific status. What is this unique theory that is well supported by scientific theory, although it still has not evidenced an experimental basis in physics?

Everett demonstrated that the choice between the particle in the one slit state and the wave in the two slit state is not necessarily an either-or situation. It is possible for both conditions to co-exist, as well as many others. The atom going through the two slit state is split into two coexisting universes, becoming branches off the world of an original universe. An observer, while recording the event, notes only the event which he, or the equipment, is capable of recording while the others continue on in their own parallel universes, unseen and unrecorded. This splitting into branching universes continually occurs every time an atom splits for any reason. Thus, there are innumerable, (ten to millions of zeros) universes that coexist simultaneously, but do not interact with each other. (A difference with light cones which, we suggested, do interact, at least on the human level.)

We are the participant observers for this one. If we wanted to try to enter another universe, we would have to go backward in time along our branch to the point where it originally bifurcated into the one we actually did enter, according to John Gribbin in his book **In Search of Schrodinger's Cat**. (In time regression in past life therapy this is exactly what is done, at least in consciousness).

Regarding choice, there is a similarity and a difference between the many-worlds and the Copenhagen interpretations. The similarity is that, in both these physics theories, deciding what he wants to observe is a choice that limits the imminent possibilities of the physicist's observations. (The collapse of the invisible quantum wave is the choice that turns it into a particle.) The difference is that the Copenhagen interpretation states that nothing else can be shown to exist prior or posterior to the exercise of a choice whereas the many worlds interpretation demonstrates that all worlds coexist on an independent reality level prior to the exercise of choice, as well as afterwards. Despite this enormous difference, both the Copenhagen interpretation and the many worlds theory are proven to be correct through quantum mechanics! Which do you choose?!

In the many worlds, it's as if, by choosing to get born into this world rather than some other one, we thereafter establish the state of physical and mental consciousness and memory of which we are aware. However, all the other possible choices that we didn't make continue on their own without our consciousness. (The quantum wave has an infinite number of possible forms until it becomes a particle.) Outrageous!

Another logical conclusion from the many worlds theory might be that we choose from the many possible states of health and illness the one that we live in currently and may have to backtrack to the point where the illness began in order to choose another one for ourselves. Actually, this would be very consistent with regressive psychotherapy which does attempt to track mental and physical illness to its first manifestations and memories, whether in past lives or in this life. In retracing the past it becomes possible to relive and abreact the pains accumulated during a past time and then reopen the options for healthier choices in current life.

The bifurcation point is also where the event or events occurred in the past that led to the choice of illness over health. It is most likely that there are many points or events, each one contributing a factor to the total 'weight' that finally leads to the choice of illness. Psychodynamically, guilt and anxiety are two of the most pernicious sources of accumulation of pain and therefore would be given the most weight on a pain scale while freedom from guilt and anxiety would be given the most weight on a pleasure scale whose end result is emotional, physical and mental health. (This should not be understood to equate having pleasure unqualifiedly as a measure of mental health).

Although the many worlds theory conflicts drastically with our commonsense ideas about how the universe works, it does not conflict, in fact it supports the methods and concepts of past life therapy and of choice as a fundamental option in life and is considered scientifically sound. The many worlds theory, choice and past life therapy are indeed strange but compatible bedfellows.

J.S.Bell constructs an interesting elaboration and support of the many worlds concept, which can be also be adopted generally psychologically and by past life regression in particular. He includes memory in the many worlds theory by developing mathematical formulae of a cosmological wave function that includes a recording device (including that of a human being, e.g. consciousness) that chooses its universe according to the "weight" of the possibilities (I called it "magnitude" earlier). The "weight" of a possibility arises out of the coherence of experienced memories. As Bell puts it,

"Everett, allowing 'A' [a memory state] to be a more complicated memory, such as that of a computer (or even a human being), or a collection of such memories, shows that only those states ... have appreciable weight in which the memories agree on a more or less coherent story of the kind we have experience of....The novelty is in the emphasis on memory contents as the essential material of physics and in the interpretation which Everett proceeds to impose on the expansion of 'E'".

"E" is a formula which includes all the information that can be recorded or "remembered" on any recording device at a certain point in time. (That would be the equivalent of point P, the present, on a light cone.) Thus Bell arrives at a formula which includes memory as part of the cosmology of quantum mechanics! [7] If we take this formula and translate it into verbal, instead of mathematical terms, it states:

(The Quantum Wave Function) x (the memory of anything, the rest of the world, and time) = (the summation of a complete set of states of the world, and the weight of a complete set of memory states) x (states of the remainder of the world and time). (Bell, 1987, P. 94)

This interpretation of Bell's E formula is probably very arguable and hypothetical, but it is presented to show that at least some physicists think there is a possibility of including consciousness in the form of memories in quantum physical math.

A cosmological wave function is needed in order to unify relativity, gravity and quantum mechanics. A cosmological wave function that includes memory is obviously not going to be acceptable to phycists, not for a long time. However, it's an integration such as that which may ultimately offer the route to the grand unified theory.

In relation to its relevance for past life regression, in Bell's opinion we do not have access to actual past events, we have only the possibility of access to memories, "and these memories are just part of the instantaneous configuration of the world" (Bell 1987 P.98).

This opens up another avenue of speculation regarding past lives. The new client coming into past life therapy asks the question whether the past life he will undergo is a fact or just a product of his imagination. The question opened up by Everett suggests the past life is real and actual, coexisting parallel to a present lifetime. Bell suggests the past life is neither a fact nor an imaginary fiction but that it is a memory of a past life retained by the subject as part of "the instantaneous configuration of the world" he lives in at present.

In other words, the branches of peoples lives follow a track through time which becomes established in a state of memory and continues along that particular track up into the present moment. It does not disappear because it is not consciously active in memory, but is evidently in some way a part of the person's world without his being aware of it. This is comparable to a fundamental assumption in past life psychotherapy, viz, that unconscious affect remaining from a past life continues somehow to communicate with contemporary events which altogether constitutes the world in which a person lives.

As noted earlier according to Everett and Gribbin, we can access earlier tracks by returning to the point in time at which that state (the past life) branched off from another life. By tracing that life down its track we can return to what are now memories of that life, but, according to Bell, not the life itself.

At the present time, this seems to be the most viable way to explain past life regression with theory in physics to give it a more scientific orientation. In this way Quontic Psychology can serve as a point from which to focus on and examine both branches of study even though they may seem so diverse as to be unrelated.

The Network of Events

There is one more step that can be taken in the application of the Many Worlds Theory, and this one returns it to its original context in physics. It will be recalled that at least 90-99% of the matter in the universe is missing and one of its explanations is called the "dark, cold matter" theory by physicists. Although they can't see it, touch it, or measure it directly, they know something more is there because they can measure gravitational pulls between the objects of visible matter such as the stars. However, the measured pull of gravitational forces cannot be adequately projected by the amount of mass of the visible matter itself. Dark matter, according to this theory, would be the dominant matter of the universe and it defines visible matter because its gravitational pull defines the shape conserving characteristics of visible matter. This dark matter is obviously primordial, it must precede in some way the appearance of gravity with its effect upon visible matter, which it is conjectured, occurred about one million years after the big bang.

Without attempting to be too mystical about it, there seems to be a case to be made for dark matter as a stuff of the universe that is not affected by the concepts of temporality, causality and locality that currently determine physical experimentation. Physicists would say they know that it must exist because of the effects of it on the visible universe but they can't say what its characterics might be because they don't have the experimental data or enough of the mathematics to describe it. Since it is not possible to define it in present-day experimental terms, physics is caught up in its own catch-22. However, if those characteristics of dark matter are considered non-linear, then it would qualify as our fifth dimension, or as Bohm's enfolded universe, or as Bell's "hidden universe" that precedes and is necessary for the visible three dimensional one to exist.

In a curious way, it could also qualify as Dirac's sea of virtual electrons, discussed in "The Purple Cow" chapter.

However, now instead of dealing with just photons and electrons, we are projecting a universe that is a sea of virtual matter of any and all kinds. As you will recall, in the description of his sea of virtual electrons, Dirac described it's relation to matter as throwing up bits of flotsam and jetsam, bits of matter popping up into existence, some remaining for awhile, others disappearing into the sea again rapidly. In other words, Dirac's sea of virtual electrons on the scale of the formation of elementary particles might very well be replicated on the scale of galaxies and universes. If so, the universe that was supposed to have begun with the Big Bang is not at all necessessarily evidence of the beginning of the universe. The Big Bang, if anything, in this view of it, was another bit of flotsam and jetsam thrown up by the sea of virtual matter, or dark matter, a visible point in an invisible ocean of a preexistent unseen universe. If you will, imagine a virtual sea of consciousness. One of virtual matter's characteristics is gravity, or something akin to gravity but it also could have an action potential that includes consciousness as well as matter of every kind.

If this is so it is most unlikely that our known universe is the only one ejected from the sea of virtual matter. It is much more likely that ours is only one of a multitude of possible, or visible universes emitted from it. Many of these other universes might continue to exist today, having changed from the virtual to the visible state unnameable light years ago prior to our own change from a virtual to a stable matter state. In that case, we would be one out of many, innumerable universes that have been born and have collapsed or died, and will die, returning to their original state in the virtual sea of dark matter after the evolutionary potential completes its course.

It is tempting to regard the Dirac sea of virtual electrons the equivalent of the sea of virtual consciousness. And Everett's Many Worlds Theory may be, in the truest sense of it, a complete theory of matter and consciousness describing the ongoing flux and flow of universe formation with beginnings and endings occurring in a matrix that is without beginning and without end.

Lao Tse knew this intuitively.

Regression in Brazil

Harmonics

I'm in a place like a mountaintop and I can see to eternity without any vision.

My consciousness is strong and knowing as a finger extending from the omniscient hand of God.

I can hear the range of all the music that was ever played without any ears.

I can speak to others, listen to their hearts and know their thoughts without any words.

I know my parents for all time and with all of memory from time immemorial.

Even though I'm not born I know all that life is because I have no existence.

— Paraphrased from a patient's experience,
D.W. Miller

The Brazilian Cultural Background

The most dramatic examples of the operation of the many worlds theory during psychotherapy happened during Organic Process sessions in Sao Paolo, Brazil. I'd gone to Sao Paolo from 1989 to 1991 to participate in the annual

International Metaphysical Conference, having conducted therapy sessions in Rio de Janeiro as well several years prior to the conference. From my work with the Brazilians, it became clear that, although many of them suffer from the same fears and blocks to accessing the fifth dimension that North Americans do, many more have already reached accessibility to paranormal levels of function. I think it's because the culture, with exceptions noted in the medical and scientific professions, generally accepts and supports contact with fifth dimensional phenomena. One sees children going to psychic healers instead of to medical doctors to heal physical as well as emotional problems, brought by their parents. Alternative forms of treatment such as acupuncture, homeopathy and spiritist psychic healing are preferred by many over medical cures. Many people acknowledge that there is value in each. Although probably more of the rich would be inclined to prefer medical treatment, I met many who subscribed to alternative forms of healing, including, of course, past life regression which was what I did there.

However, it sometimes turned out that what I thought would be a past life regression took on other forms that I did not anticipate and had not encountered in my work with European/American people. The following are a couple of examples of the turns that sessions took in Sao Paolo. I think they are fine examples of the principles that I have been describing in the rest of this book.

The Case of the Fearful Shaman

His jerky, nervous movements, wide dark eyes darting bird-like around the room beneath a neatly groomed, wavy head of black hair bespoke anxiety underneath his clean, pressed clothing. When I asked for a voluteer in the group in Sao Paolo to do a past life regression I knew I would probably choose him if he showed any kind of openness to the process. For one thing, he spoke English fluently so I wouldn't need a Portugese translation. In speaking to the group about himself he revealed that he had images that frightened him - images of being in strange countries that he never actually visited, like Egypt. He had had spiritual experiences, he thought, since the age of four. Sometimes an impulse came, he couldn't trace it's source, that took him out of his body and frightened him. He'd return suddenly, like dropping down with a thump back into his body. He liked people and knew he wanted to help them but thought he needed some help himself.

I'd observed him enter the workshop room about an hour late with a stout, light-skinned, un-Brazilian looking woman who said she read Tarot. She said his problem was that he was too good to others, he would give too much of himself away and they took advantage of him. She was obviously a strong supporter.

I felt that his energy was probably the most available for a regression so, when he volunteered, I chose him for the demonstration.

He lay down on the royal purple 5' by 8' rug covering the foam rubber, followed instructions to breathe deeply and in relaxing his body into the trance state I could see that he rapidly entered deeper layers of the unconscious. His body began twitching uncontrollably with a fairly regular pattern centered around his feet, a pulse was visibly pounding in his stomach near the diaphragm and his lips were moving though nothing was audible.

The dialogue that follows is not verbatim but is very close to what occurred. "FS" stands for "Fearful Shaman" and "DM" stands for myself.

DM: What are you feeling?
FS: Frightened, very frightened.
DM: What are you seeing?
FS: Nothing, nothing.
DM: Nothing?
FS: Just a vague form.

DM: O.K. Let's go slowly. Let it take a shape.
FS: Yes, it's forming something.
DM: Yes? (pause for an answer, nothing forthcoming) Is it a person?
FS: I can't tell. (pause) Yes, perhaps.

I thought that we had very quickly reached a past life figure, but it turned out that we had not. The person that he saw was his father in his present life. He was there to block his path and to prevent him from going any further into the past. I realized that I had neglected to do my usual inquiry about relationships with parents in this life by asking for information and memories that would help establish the continuity between the past life and problems in the current life. However, the priorities reasserted themselves anyway. As I inquired about his present life experiences, particularly in relation to parents, I realized that he was coming out of the trance state, but continued anyway because I thought the information was important.

His father had always been a very distant person with whom he'd had very little contact even though he never left the family. He felt neither anger nor love toward his father. He was essentially a non-entity in his life. He had died approximately three years ago and he had no feelings about his death. I briefly challenged his lack of feeling about his father, but felt that his defenses were too hardened to deal with in this session. I hoped we could get around them. He had been raised by his mother with whom he shared loving feelings (probably Oedipally, but didn't go into that).

I didn't want to lose the trance state completely so with just that sketchy family biography I asked him whether he could return to the relaxed state. He said he thought he could. He lay down, breathed deeply again, and after a few minutes the leg movements and the diaphragm pulse returned. I asked him to see his father again and to ask him to leave. He did so. He told him he had no right to block his path. His father resisted leaving, claimed his right to do what he thought best for his son, but finally complied with his son's request. I asked him to continue breathing deeply, to allow himself to sink more deeply into his body and to return to the entrance to the past life. His body continued the involuntary twitch and when, after awhile, I asked whether he was in the past yet, he said he was. Was his father present? No, he was not. What could he see? He could see another figure forming.

DM: Can you see his feet? Can you see what he is wearing? Just tell me whatever you can see.
       The pulse in his diaphragm was vibrating rhythmically and fast, legs were moving in and out, side to side, and breathing was deep and regular.

FS: Yes, it's forming - a man -strange clothing - dark skin, thin, like in India.

DM: Yes? What else is there?

FS: He is alone.

As he became clearer, the man's personality also started to take shape. He was an Eastern Indian, well-dressed, of some special status in that society. He was a spiritual man and appeared to be clothed in flowing religious garments. As the description of the man grew sharper and stronger, FS became more agitated. His body movements became more spasmodic and his breathing became laborious. It was evident that he was becoming more frightened.

DM: Who is this man?

FS: I don't know. He's a spiritual man.

DM: What are you feeling?

FS: I'm frightened, very frightened.

DM: Tell me about your fear.

FS: I don't want to be him.

DM: No? Why not? Why don't you want to be him?

FS: He is an important person. He is somebody special. I don't want to be somebody special.

DM: How can you tell that he is somebody special?

FS: There are many people around him. They expect
       something of him. He is a very spiritual man.
DN: Can you tell what country you are in? Do you know?
FS: I can't tell for sure. From the clothes they're wearing,
       Egypt maybe.
DM: What do they expect of him?
FS: There is a fire.
DM: There is a fire?
FS: Yes.
DM: Where? Is the house burning? Is it in a fireplace?
FS: It is in a box.
DM: In a box? (My confusion must have been very plain.)
FS: Yes. He is being given the fire by an old man. The
       old man is someone special too.

I quickly decided to accept the irrationality of "a fire in a
box" since it appeared to be a religious rite.

DM: Why is he being given the fire in the box?
FS: He is one of them now. He is a spiritual leader of the
       people. He has done many good things for them. He
       doesn't want to be a leader, but he is.
DM: What are they saying to him?
FS: It is in a strange language, but I can understand it
       somehow.
DM: Can you speak it now?
FS: No. It's Hebrew. I don't know Hebrew.

I made a mental note of the shift in identity from Indian
to Egyptian to Hebrew and decided not to challenge it at
present. Either way, it was a strange country with a strange
language and I didn't think that the consistency and logic of
it was the most important thing. Perhaps it would be possible
later to verify the fire in the box ritual as a spiritual rite in
either culture.

He next described a scene in which he in turn was handing
over the fire in the box to someone else. He was now older,

and this was a younger man who would help him in his work.

It had been over an hour already, I felt we had a fairly long ways to go to resolve this experience and I sensed the group was getting restless and losing interest, though I was intensely involved. I asked whether he knew the name of the spiritual man, but he didn't know it, nor the exact century in which the event was taking place. Later I thought that the shift from an Egyptian to a Hebrew culture, though confusing at first, may have indicated a time period that scaled the flight from Egypt to the early period of the Hebrew nation. There is also sometimes, especially in early regression sessions, pressure from different past lives as if several want to come in at once and there is a consequent shift in identification of various elements in the story. However, I didn't want to shift him into a logical mode because it would seriously interfere with the story line which itself appeared cohesive and consistent.

In order to complete a session I invariably request the person to envisage the death of the person in that lifetime, to tell me how and where it occurs, under what circumstances, whether illness or natural death, an accident or whatever, and so on with as many details as possible. When I asked for information about the manner of death of the religious leader, FS's body abruptly began shaking in great agitation and he began to cry.

FS: No, I don't want to.
DM: No? Why not? Is it too terrible to see?
FS: Yes. I don't want to see it.
DM: I understand, but it is very important for you to see it. This seems to be a strong cause of your fear. It will help to release you from your fear if you can let yourself see it, and experience your death in that life.
FS: Alright. (He regains control of himself and his body stops shaking.)
DM: Tell me what happens. How do you die?
FS: I am asleep in my bed and I am murdered.

DM: How are you murdered?
FS: With a knife.

I note that in order to relate the event he has to avoid his emotions so has detached himself. He has become factual and rational.

DM: Please start at the very beginning. Take it one step at a time. What are the circumstances? Go slowly up to the moment of death itself and experience it as fully as you can.

FS: I am in my bed, asleep. I can feel him in my room. It is dark so I can't see him. I know that he wants to kill me.

DM: Why does he want to kill you? Who is he?

FS: He is my first assistant, but he is jealous of me (quiet sobbing).

DM: He's jealous of you?

FS: He is jealous of my power and of my standing among the people.

DM: What does he want?

FS: He wants power for himself.

DM: Is he doing this alone, or is he part of a group?

FS: A group. It's another sect, a sect that wants to have more power. He is the leader of that sect.

DM: What do you feel?

FS: I want him to kill me. I am waiting for him. I can see him now.

The intensity of his crying increases.

DM: Yes? And what happens next?

FS: (He is obviously very frightened but accepts the inevitability of the murder without resistance. He struggles, puts his hand on his diaphragm and breathes heavily as if struggling for air. He thrashes about uncontrollably, then his body gradually grows calmer, his breathing becomes steady and easy.)

DM: What's happening?

FS: I can see my soul, my spirit (his voice has a questioning intonation)? It seems to be over me now. But it isn't me. It is me and it isn'tme.

DM: (I'm a little confused by this because it is usually clear which is body and which is spirit.) What do you mean?

FS: There's my spirit but its not me, it's like somebody else's spirit.

DM: It's not the spirit of the spiritual leader?

FS: Yes, but it's not me.

DM: (I develop a sense that he's talking from his present self.) Are you in your present body?

FS: Yes.

This is not the way it usually happens. The spirit of the dead person does not hover over the present person but over the body of the deceased.

DM: Do you mean he is here in present time?

FS: Yes, he's here.

DM: Why is he here? What does he want of you?

FS: He wants to give me instruction. He wants to direct me on the right path.

D: OK. But he belongs to the world of the other spirits.

FS: No, he doesn't want to go there. He wants to stay here to instruct me.

DM: Is he like your spiritual guide?

FS: Yes.

DM: Do you want him to remain as your spiritual guide?

FS: I don't know.

DM: You have a choice here. He doesn't have to remain if you don't want him to. Although he is a very powerful entity you have the power to make him go if you want him to.

FS: (long silence, no answer)

DM: Do you want him to stay?

FS: Yes.

DM: Do you want him to guide you on your spiritual path?

FS: Yes.

DM: You can do that if you want to, you can let him stay. But he had a terrible death. He was murdered. People who have been murdered, or commit suicide, often either don't realize they are dead or they don't want to leave the earthly plane. They're not ready to go because of the circumstances around their death. A part of you is afraid to go on the spiritual path because of what happened to him.

FS: Yes, I know about that now.

DM: Since he was murdered and he was your own past life you carry in you the fear of his death happening again on your own spiritual path.

FS: Yes, I don't want that.

DM: But this is also a new life. You can do it differently this time. That fear doesn't really belong to you now in this life. Can you separate that fear that belongs to him in the past life from you present life to go on without it?

FS: Yes, I want to do that.

DM: OK. You may continue to need help with that. But he is a very powerful spiritual leader, he has a lot to teach you and it's worth a try. Later on, you many need some help again. Are you ready to return fully to your present body?

FS: Yes.

DM: OK. I'll count slowly backwards from 20 to 1 and when I'm finished you will be fully present in the here and now, in your present body, in this room, fully in your own life. Are you ready?

FS: Yes.

When I finish counting, he opens his eyes. They are steady, his body is resting quietly, he looks around, and then at me.

DM: Are you fully here?
FS: Yes. But I'm very tired.
DM: Would you rather talk to the people here now, or would you rather rest quietly in a private room?
FS: Privately.

I take him to a room and make him comfortable. We chat a bit. He is feeling fine, the anxiety is not evident. In his discussion with the group later he shows that he has recalled and fully grasped what has happened during the session. He understands the implication of keeping the spiritual guide with him and that it means he is committed to his spiritual path. I support his purpose and assure him that he has a great deal of spiritual ability which is well worth developing. We part company and I am not sure that I will ever see him again since I'm leaving Brazil the next day.

Isadora and the Inca

On Thursday, June 6, 1991 at 9:00 A.M., working in the Pax Center in Sao Paolo, I found out that the client for that hour had cancelled and, having too many clients to see that day, I had no regrets. At 9:15 I was told by an interpreter that a woman with an appointment with another therapist had seen Gular interviewing me on his TV show and insisted on having a session with me. Gular was the erstwhile Johnny Carson of Brazil.

It was the beginning of the strangest contact with another person that I've ever had. I'd come down to Sao Paolo for the third year in a row to deliver a paper about homeostasis and quontic psychology at the Fourth International Metaphysical Conference. It was my sixth trip to Brazil. After the conference came plans for the TV show, newspaper interviews, and a weekend workshop. My sessions in Organic Process/Past Life Therapy took hold and I was much in demand. However, someone trying to break the door down because it was urgent for her to see me was unusual.

After some discussion with an interpreter, I agreed to talk to her to find out why it was so important for her to see me rather than the other therapist who had been assigned to her. She entered my office, not over five feet tall, rotund, with dark skin and black hair, wearing an unattractive dress. In Portugese (she spoke no English) she said she had received "a message" (from a spirit was implied) saying that she was supposed to see a past life therapist and when she saw me on Gular's program she said "that's him". Perhaps more out of curiosity than anything else, I agreed to give up my free time to work with her.

I conducted the usual questioning period that I use to find out what problems exist in the here and now of a person's life. This will help later to establish the continuity between past and present problems. She said that she didn't have big problems, only little things here and there that she could manage by herself and that she was happy enough with her husband and her children. I assumed that I was being given the standard defensive maneuver of "I'm not going to take responsibility for myself by telling you anything, but perform a magic feat and heal me of everything immediately with one past life regression".

However, further inquiry about her present life and her childhood did not reveal anything traumatic or even very painful. She described her childhood as one in which she had enough freedom to make her own choices and to enjoy herself. She came from Bolivia where the family wasn't well off, but had enough for ongoing needs. I could not locate very strong blocks against feelings, she seemed honest and open enough. I then decided that I didn't have to wait for a second session, as I usually do, to conduct a regression.

During the relaxation to induce a trance state, her breathing was deep and more relaxed, without fear, than I expected. However, as the relaxation procedure, which starts with the feet, proceeded toward her head her breathing became very labored and she made sounds that seemed to come from a great and difficult depth. I wondered whether she had entered a birth primal, which is usually very stressful, but as I listened further I felt she was in a deeply unconscious trance state. I asked her to tell me what she was experiencing but she only continued her intense breathing while making deep sounds. I considered the possibility that she had become a medium for a spirit entity.

As an exploration of that idea, I invited an entity to make itself known and to speak to Isadora. Her breathing became more labored, as if she were becoming very anxious. I thought I was on the right track and reassured the entity that we were its friend and would not harm it. We just wanted to make contact. Almost inaudibly, in a deep voice, it said, "I'm here".

The following section, which is not verbatim from the audio tape, is a summary of the interactions that occurred as I recalled them on the following day. This is followed by a section which is more audible which is close as possible to verbatim. The second day is again a summary. "DM" stands for my inquiries and "SE" stands for Spirit Entity. When she speaks, an "I" will stand for Isadora. The session lasted over an hour and a half.

After the entity announced its presence I addressed it.

DM: Why have you come to visit Isadora?
SE: I've come because she is one of us.
DM: Who are you?
SE: There are many of us here.
DM: Can you tell me where you are from?
SE: We are from Maachu Pichu.
DM: Why are you here? Why are you still connected to an earth person, a human being with flesh and blood?
SE: She is one of us.
DM: What do you mean? Who are you?
SE: We are Inca.
DM: You are Inca?
SE: We are guardians of Maachu Pichu and Porto do Sol.
DM: Why have you come to visit her?
SE: There is much that we want her to know. They have caused us great suffering.

DM: Who has caused you suffering?
SE: The people of flesh and blood who have come and destroyed us and our places. But we are still here. We guard our temples.

Later, I realized that I was puzzled by this destruction and its timing, but didn't pursue it. It's possible that as entities that died in a terrible way centuries ago under the Spaniards, they didn't go on to prepare for another life but have remained at Maachu Pichu to protect it from other ravaging humans. He may not be aware of the human quality of time.

DM: What do you want Isadora to do?
SE: She must come back.
DM: Where must she come back to?
SE: She must come back to Maachu Pichu where she is from.
DM: What must she do there?
SE: She must tell other humans of flesh and blood about us. She must tell them about us.
DM: That you are the guardians?
SE: Yes, that we guard the temples and the secret places. She must know this.
DM: What is your name?
SE: (There is a long pause, then a period of stuttering and reiteration of a "Ka, Ka, Ka" and a long "O" and an expirated "Ah" which sounded to me like Kakakakoah).
DM: Kakakakoah?
SE: (The name was repeated again laboriously. It sounded like Kakooah and I decided to let it go at that.)

The following section is transcribed as closely as possible from the tape recording.

DM: What must Isadora do when she comes back to Maachu Pichu?
SE: In the area of the earth -where you see the silver snow on the mountain - The energy is a strong force.

DM: The snow is?

SE: That's why it never disappears, the snow. This place throws the energy (translation problem)

DM: ...throws the energy everywhere?

SE: Yes, the snow never melts. It is a very important point of energy. It throws the energy into the air.

DM: This is a very special kind of energy?

SE: Yes. You will feel its power.

DM: Can you tell me something about your relationship to her?

SE: I send her to do something. For her to have knowledge with human beings. I was the one who sent her and sometime she has to come back.

DM: Back where?

SE: To the place where she belongs, she has to come back.

DM: Where does she have to come back to?

SE: To Maachu Pichu. Within her body she doesn't know..

DM: She doesn't know?

SE: She doesn't know these places that I am talking about. She has to know all those places that I am talking about. She has to go there.

DM: OK. Why?

SE: Because she has to know. With the eye she has to look at the Porto do Sol that nobody has known yet.

DM: Is that the Golden Door?

SE: (translator's difficulty gives me the impression it is in Maachu Pichu which becomes corrected through SE). No, it is the Porto do Sol in Bolivia. She has to know this place. In Tihuanaco.

DM: Tiajuan...is in Bolivia?

SE: It's in Bolivia.

DM: Where in Bolivia? Please tell her clearly. So she'll know where it is.

SE: Tihuanaco.

DM: Tihuanaco. OK.

SE: She has to look at this place. There is the reason for our relationship. And then she will know about ourselves. In this place is written something.

DM: Something is written?

SE: She will realize what has happened between us.

DM: Meaning between who and who?

SE: (translator) Between he and she.

DM: Are you somebody she has known in a past life? Why did you choose her?

SE: I knew she will do everything that I tell her to do, and she would understand.

DM: Understand what?

SE: There is a door that leads to a staircase, deep underground. It has a secret inscription and she must read what it says. It is very important for her to know what the inscription says.

DM: Why is it important?

SE: I am forbidden to tell. It is a secret. She must decode the inscription around the door.

DM: But if it is a secret how can she decode it?

SE: She must read it. She will know how to read it.

DM: (I still don't get the location of the Porto do Sol.) The Porto do Sol is in Maachu Pichu?

SE: No. Porto do Sol is different. Porto do Sol is in Tihuanaco. It is in Bolivia.

DM: Porto do Sol is in Bolivia? Then why must she go to Maachu Pichu? Do you live in Maachu Pichu or in Porto do Sol?

SE: Lake Titicaca was made by Inca. We live deep under the waters of Lake Titicaca. But we also protect Porto Do Sol.

DM: Why is it important to go to Maachu Pichu?

SE: In Maachu Pichu there is a door to a staircase. This staircase leads to a secret city. There is a secret city under Maachu Pichu. We used to live there, now we live deep in Lake Titicaca.

DM: How will she know where to find the staircase?

SE: She must go there and she will know. We appear as lights and we will be able to help her.

I recalled my long unfulfilled desire to visit the Inca ruins at Maachu Pichu ever since my Egyptian physicist friend had said "Aventura" and I had seen this word over a description of Maachu Pichu.

DM: Do I have some kind of connection to all this? Do you have any knowlege of me, do you have any connection with me?

SE: (pause and heavy breathing) Yes. You are a brother, one of my brothers, from the same civilization. He chose you.

DM: (I controlled my skepticism). Is there anything you want me to do?

SE: I want you to help us through her. Help her to have more knowledge. Go there to know the place. Look at it. She will know why we are going to be together. Look into the Porto do Sol. I want us to help the people there, the human beings around.

DM: Do you want to stay around her, or is it possible you can leave her?

SE: I need to tell her - but first I need to tell someone else, I need to talk to my brothers first, but she will feel me very close to her, together, Daniel. (She is weeping.)

DM: I feel very close to you also. I have had a wish to go to Maachu Pichu.

SE: It is needed that you come back.

DM: Tell me what I can do when I go there, how I can serve.

SE: Daniel - it has to do with Porto Do Sol. You are going to see what is written there. You are going to find out something. You have to see all the details that is there.

DM: All the details? In Porto do Sol? (pause - it's getting late for the next session so I have to end it) I thank you very much for coming to speak to us. We will try to contact you again. Is it OK now for us to part from each other?

SE: Yes, its OK. (translation problem) I am afraid of human beings - I am not afraid -.

DM: Do you know that we are your friends and we will stay in contact with you. Adios. I am now going to count to twenty. When I finish counting she will return fully to her own body in this room.

I: I am lying there, nobody sees me. I am lying there on the mountain. I want to stay there. It is very beautiful.

DM: I agree that it is very beautiful for you to be there but you are obliged to be in your body, for now. And with your knowledge and your wisdom you will be able to help the Inca people, so it is necessary now to return to your body. Are you ready to return?

I: (she is unwilling to return)

DM: You will not be able to help, do you understand?

I: Yes.

DM: Are you ready to return now?

I: Yes.

DM: OK. So I will start counting to twenty and when I am done you will be fully in your body.

I'd worked with other people who didn't want to return and knew that the attraction of the fifth dimension was overpowering. Insisting seemed to be the only thing that worked. After I brought her back to present time and place, since it was forceful, I was concerned about how she felt, but there was nothing to be alarmed about. She was happy to have made the contact, her affect was cheerful as we discussed another appointment to channel the Inca again in a couple of days. This time she said she didn't want to pay the fee because it would be for my benefit. (Very much in touch with reality, I thought.) I agreed to split it with her since it was for the benefit of both of us. She would return on Monday, the morning of my departure from Sao Paolo.

I felt the coincidence of Isadora showing up at a time when another session had been cancelled, with a connection with

Maachu Pichu that had more than casual significance for me. It might be a synchronistic merging of three dimensional and fifth dimensional energies in my own life as well as in Isadora's. It felt as if a resonance phenomena, which will be elaborated later, had taken place. My own reference to a channelled experience that I had with a spirit entity went back around twenty years to Jean Louis Cattaui. (See the Winter 1990 issue of VOICES published by the American Academy of Psychotherapists - Miller 1990.) He had left me with the word"Aventura" which obviously meant adventure. I saw the word spelled out just as he had pronounced it many years later, six years ago, as the banner of an inside page in a Rio de Janeiro newspaper, during my first trip to Brazil to conduct therapy sessions. Under the banner was a description of Maachu Pichu and I thought that this might have been what my friend meant. Nevertheless, I suppose I wasn't convinced enough to follow through on the message. And now comes Isadora. Sometimes, I know I need a push. I told her I would like to go to Maachu Pichu, possibly next year, but I didn't yet know whether I could arrange it.

For the second session, the trance induction was brief. Isadora made contact with the Inca after just a few minutes of relaxation. His voice came through more deeply and firmly than before. I acknowledged the strength of his presence. I wanted to clear up the uncertainty about his name. This time it came through without the alliterated "Ka" as "Karooa" with a heavily accented "aaah" at the end. I asked him to spell it. I gave Isadora a pen and paper and without opening her eyes she painstakingly wrote his name. I remarked that there was a "k" in the middle, sounding like "Kakooah". He said it could also be spelled "roa", which she wrote on a second line, and that either way was acceptable. Verbally, however he always pronounced it "Karooah" with the "r", though he apparently spelled it with a "k". I know nothing about Inca language. He said something about having a different language than the one we speak, presumably Inca.

I asked him whether he knew that we were hoping to come to Maachu Pichu and Porto do Sol, maybe next year. He said he did. The following is according to my recall, since the tape was blurry, a short time later.

DM: I am looking forward to the trip.
SE: Yes. I will appear to you in Maachu Pichu.
DM: You will appear to me? (very startled) How?
SE: I will appear as a light.
DM: As a light? But how will I know you from other lights?

I could feel myself tense up.

SE: I will come close to you. Do not be afraid.
DM: Alright. I will look for you. I won't be afraid.
SE: You will have a very strong experience, you will experience a very strong energy.
DM: O.K. I'm looking forward to meeting you.
SE: Good. I will go now.
DM: Until then.

At the end, Isadora was in good spirits, if you know what I mean, and both of us were hoping to meet again in Maachu Pichu. As of this writing, the trip to Maachu Pichu and Porto do Sol has not yet occurred and my attempt to contact the people in Brazil to make plans has not been successful. I'm frustrated and disappointed but still hope to meet Karooah one day.

Part III

How to Receive Messages from the Future Before They Are Sent

Symmetry and its Breaking, or,
Is Dr. Weinberg Listening?

"At birth, the universe was exceedingly hot and existed in a state of perfect unbroken symmetry...Some of the symmetry relations between forces and particles broke...(and) the universe degenerated from a phase containing unified forces and identical particles to the modern, more familiar state of differing forces and particles."

— Spergel & Turock 1992 [1]

The Chess Game

The paradox of the Newtonian laws of causality with its focus on determinism and predictability butting against the quantum law of uncertainty with its focus on indeterminism and statistical alternatives explaining the same reality can be resolved if the laws of nature are seen analogously to a game of chess.

In a game of chess there are certain rules that make up a game which provide causal action-response effects. Move a piece into a certain square covered by the opponent's piece, whose range of movement is determined by the rules of the game, and that first piece can be removed by the second. This is a cause-effect response based on rules created to govern a locally determined environment. However, viewed on a larger scale, the first player has a great deal of choice about which piece he will move, just as the second player has. Depending on his experience in playing the game, his acuity perceptually, his problem-solving intelligence, the first player may or may not choose to move into the set of squares in which his piece can be removed by the other player's piece. The second player as well may not decide to remove the first player's piece, seeing a trap for a more valuable piece as a more favorable move.

Each player moving a piece affects the entire layout of the board as well as those pieces closest to him. There are consequently two levels at which the game is played at the board. Any movement will have a larger effect upon the total interactions of the arrangement of the pieces on the board and in particular there will be local consequences of any particular action. Choices made at the local level ultimately affects what will happen to every piece on the board—and both players affect further choices and interactions. The players themselves are crucial to determining the outcome of the game and any action alters the effects and the possibilities of other pieces further removed from the immediate action just as much as it affects the probabilities of the fate of a particular chesspiece.

Rules are obviously created by people who invent games such as chess. These rules, passed on to subsequent players, become the information base on which the game is played. Thus there grows a stable part of the game which the inheritance of information repeatedly reinforces until it appears as if those rules are totally inclusive and final even while it leaves much room for alternative possibilities, choices of movement, for all the pieces which the game's rules have placed on the board. Once established, the rules are seldom if ever changed, even though they could be.

There are, according to the state vector and the particle-wave dilemma, an innumerable variety of kinds of games which can be made to appear on the board, which is ulti-mately the statement of Everett's Many Worlds Theory. The board, the pieces and the information are Nature's, God's, Brahma's, or The Inconceivable One's contribution to the game. Newtonian science says that the rules as well are made up by nature which has set laws by which the pieces function. Now quantum physicists are daring to suggest that the rules may be made up by the players and the board and pieces are selectively chosen from an innumerable set of options provided by nature.

In any language, the depth at which you understand the game will provide you with information that will determine how (that is, according to what rules) and how well you move your pieces and, in turn, that set of circumstances will determine the outcome of the game. The game is not determined either by "fate" or by "chance". It is determined by choices selected out of many probabilities within a set of given possibilities whose actual existence is indeterminate until they are ultimately perceived as structures. The more possibilities a person sees, the greater variety of structures he can create, until the rules are set. (This is the condition with which evolution operates, going from possibilities to structures, which become set up into rules of nature.) Then, the better he understands his choices within those rules the better he can play the game. And the more moves he has made in the past, the more effective will his resources be within his store of memories to choose the most successful move.

Thus, the creation of the universe as we know it can be perceived as such a "move", made by "Nature" or "Brhama" or "God" or "The Big Bang" or "The Homeostatic Principle" out of its own dynamics. However, how far can we go in this metaphor for life as being indeterminate until choices of some kind are made? Did we, as an intrinsic part of the dynamics of the universe, participate in creating the equivalent of the big bang? If that's the way the universe actually began, it would mean that life is a move in which we ourselves in some form or other have participated at the outset and are continuing to participate in its evolution by virtue of our choices.

How far and what meaning does this question of choice have in our lives? Did choice enter in for humans only after we developed into conscious beings through evolutionary processes? Or was it some all-powerful being, a God, doing it all while we were and still are the outcome of His actions and wishes, as conventional religion has it, and have nothing but moral choices to make? If we did participate at the very start was it through sharing with some form of consciousness in the energy that makes the universe what it is and was it a passive sharing or an active participation in the choice itself? If that is the case, that we shared actively in making first choices, then do we in this universe, in this consciousness, exist in fact on the chessboard of our lives in such a way as to continually affect the structures in which we live with the same awesome powers?

And, most significantly, are there not other kinds of universes with other kinds of information as structural determinants which we don't actually have available in this particular universe? Can we ever know anything at all about them? Just what constitutes our possibilities for knowledge and what constitutes our finite, unbridgeable limits? Have we arrived at them yet?

The search for knowledge about ourselves and about the universe we inhabit itself may have affected the course of our evolution, for better and for worse. However, in general, I feel optimistic about man's durability. In Evolution, the "moves" are those in favor of survival, the "memories" are the genetic structures that develop into resources for survival. The game moves in the direction of a homeostasis achieved by the continuation of the game and its continuation is the way that we win it.

The Symmetry Group of Nature

Does physics have anything in particular to offer to the homeostatic principle which is so relevant to quontic psychology and implicitly to the other sciences? The search for a Grand Unified Theory can be interpreted as a search for such a principle. In the process, physicists have developed a particular set of concepts with mathematical support for their own variation on homeostasis. Recently, that is within the past ten years or so, Steven Weinberg at the University of Texas and Abdul Salaam at Princeton University have been working on and have shared a Nobel Prize for their work on "the symmetry group of nature".

It is usually acknowledged that quantum mechanics is an extraordinarily accurate mathematical description of atomic operations whose causes and purposes are not understood. It constitutes a stage with mechanical operations without any actors, actions without definable conditions created by an author that makes the actions take the course that they do. As Weinberg points out, the actions of quantum mechanics needs a principle. This principle may be supplied by the concept that he helped to develop, the concept of symmetry. This, we will find, is the contribution that physics makes to the principle of homeostasis, which we have pointed out is common ground accepted by all the sciences we have looked at so far, individually within their own restricted areas of study. Well then, what is symmetry in quantum mechanics?

In physics it does not have the same meaning and usage as it does in everyday English. To quote Weinberg about the state vector (See Figure 14., *State Vector*, on page 128.):

> "A symmetry principle is a statement that there are various ways that you can change the way you look at nature, which actually changes the direction the state vector is pointing, but which do not change the rules that govern how the state vector rotates with time. The set of all these changes of point of view is called the symmetry group of nature. It is increasingly clear that the symmetry group of nature is the deepest thing that we understand about nature today. I would

like to suggest something here that I am not really certain about but which is at least a possibility: that specifying the symmetry group of nature may be all we need to say about the physical world, beyond the principle of quantum mechanics." (Weinberg 1987)[2] (Weinberg 1992)[3]

In our own way of recapitulating this statement, Weinberg says that even though we are focusing our kaleidoscope on a different pattern of events in nature, we are not actually doing anything that changes the fundamental rules of nature. These stable rules governing how things work, no matter what changes are imposed by the perceiver upon any of the phenomena he may be capable of turning to are collectively called the symmetry group of nature. They take place at the deepest level of understanding of which we are capable today.

There is the level of choice as well, represented by the state vector which may point in a direction determined by the particular direction that you, the actor on the system, may want it to take. There are certain stable rules about the way it changes which are fixed, but its possibilities are not fixed.

Underneath the state vector which may change its position by rotating in time and point in a different direction there is a basic principle which will keep it attuned to functioning within the set of rules governing the workings of natural phenomena. This basic principle representing both stability and change is the symmetry group of nature in physics. It is the physics version of the chess game.

Symmetry in quantum physics is also one special aspect of the more general principle of homeostasis in quontic psychology which is seen to govern organic as well as inorganic matter. Physics, by the nature of its concerns, does not investigate or theorize about organic matter. It dismisses organic matter as a separate field even if it is worthy of study, since it too is made up of atoms and molecules. However, organic matter follows some different rules with modes of operation providing for different kinds of functions than non-organic matter. The rules for organic matter include such functions as self-determined mobility, growth processes dependent on sunlight and air, consciousness and choice - so physics can never claim to explain more than its own special, limited area of investigation and should stop claiming to explain everything possible. The symmetry group is a wonderful philosophic as well as mathematical concept, but it will not explain everything as Weinberg claims until it can be shown how it can be applied to organic as well as inorganic life.

The quotation at the head of this chapter brings our book full circle. When I first constructed the diagram called "Synchronistic Perception in a Fragmented State" (Figure 2) I had not read much, if anything, of Weinberg's formulation of symmetry and had understood even less of it. Now, about four years later, symmetry brings the diagram back with new meaning and added significance.

It turns out that physics too has a pendulum that swings between synchronistic, wholistic or unified states and a fragmented state. The synchronistic state in the upper half of the diagram is called unbroken symmetry and the fragmented state in the lower half is called broken symmetry in physics. Symmetry is used by Weinberg in a general sense to describe the rules operating the functions of the universe while others use it to describe the earliest steps that led to the creation of the universe as we know it. Either way, the concept of symmetry breaking runs back to back with symmetry, just as fragmentation does in relation to the synchronistic state.

In its state of unbroken symmetry, all the known particles and all four forces that bind particles together were integrated and functioned as a single state. "These symmetries, which become evident in experiments conducted at high-energy particle accelerators, would similarly have been exposed in the first moments of the universe." (Spergel and Turok 1992, P. 55)

Although such experiments confirm the fragmentation of energy, only theoretical and mathematical speculation supports the unbroken symmetry theory. Particle accelerators still can't produce unbroken symmetry any more than they can produce unbroken consciousness or unbroken homeostasis. I think it is futile to suppose they ever will. We may speculate ad infinitum about the rules that existed preceding the creation of the universe - and mankind has done a great deal of it beginning for us in the West with the story of creation in the Bible - but to physically recreate creation would destroy the universe and return it to its uncreated state. Then we would know and would have the ultimate physics experiment in which we would have proven the Grand Unified Theory, but there would be nobody around to tell it to because everyone would be blissed out in unbroken symmetry. Actually, it might be something to look forward to. Dr. Weinberg, are you listening?

At the level of first principles functioning in the universe I find Dr. Weinberg supports the homeostatic principle in the following statement:

> "...At the deepest level, all we find are symmetries and responses to symmetries. Matter itself dissolves, and the universe itself is revealed as one large reducible representation of the symmetry group of nature".

Despite its own conceptual limitations imposed by it's scientific experimental structure, the symmetry group may be broadened, in effect, to wipe out the differences between organic and inorganic processes and relate to a basic metaphysical principle which underlies both once again. Of course good physicists reject any metaphysical or paranormal implications in anything they say but it is not likely that the symmetry group of nature will manifest itself in concrete data except as an implication. Nevertheless, the implications of its presence are everywhere, in the manifestation of everything that happens and not least of all in quantum physics. Don't tell any physicists that they are metaphysicians, but I think "the ineluctable one" of Buddhist philosophy has won the scientific day again.

Scalar Waves and Further Dynamics in the Quontic Loop

"Space is merely a relation between two sets of data, and an infinite number of times may coexist. Here and there, past and present, are relative, not absolute, and change according to the ordinates and coordinates selected. Observational science has in fact led back to the purest subjective idealism...."

— R.W. Clark, Einstein [1]

Soliton Biomedics

It has been proposed that more than physically ascertainable, perhaps more esoteric, fifth dimensional dynamics might be integral to the memory process. We have proposed that there is a metaphysical aspect of memory that might conceivably interact with the physical aspect in some way and that these two levels influence each other. Is any research on that possibility available?

Electrons and therefore electromagnetic fields are undoubtedly responsible for some part of the mechanisms involving memory storage and transmission in everyday life. Recent research by Dr. Glen Rein, biomedical research biologist at Stanford University Medical Center, also supports the extension of those functions into the paranormal domain. For example, he states,

"...these [Tesla Waves] nonlinear fields do not decay with time or distance from their source and therefore do not lose their energy or information content upon transmission. Furthermore, they can travel faster than the speed of light and since they exist in complex four dimensional space, they can change the rate of flow of time, thereby giving them rather paranormal properties...." (Rein 1988[2])

These waves are also commonly referred to as scalar waves or as solitons. A soliton is a wave that retains its shape over unusually long distances and does not dissipate. It evidently runs contrary to the second law of thermodynamics, which states that the universe drifts toward increasing disorder, or entropy; thus, the universe will eventually run down and collapse into itself. It states that some energy gets lost in any use of energy, like car fuel in which some is used and some is sent to the exhaust as waste. "Yet solitons exist, and by rolling along indefintely they seem to defy the inexorable trend toward entropy", according to Scott (1990). [3]

Rein also describes how cell membranes of organisms are non-linear and are capable of conduction via bioelectromagnetic waves using solitons as carriers of information. These same non-linear bioelectromagnetic waves have been found to exist in the cellular activity of the nervous system. In <u>The Sciences</u>, journal of the N.Y. Academy of Sciences, Scott reports:

"Physical scientists and mathematicians are beginning to suspect that microspcopic solitons can traverse the cell. Neurologists have begun to understand that nerve impulses travel from the brain to the hand just as a soliton crosses the ocean [without losing energy, like a tidal wave]. And knowledge of solitons is being applied to one

of the fundamental mysteries of biology:
How is energy converted from one form to
another in living organisms?"(Scott 1990 [4])

The soliton wave is not restricted in size or location and travels just as efficiently in outer space as it does in neurological space. It is a form of energy which apparently is now being corroborated through biomedical research just as it had been in physical and electromagnetic research. It's role in each is not clear, but the possibilities are extremely inviting.

In Rein's research, scalar waves are also considered to be possible mediators for self-healing and transpersonal healing phenomena. We have also been suggesting that acausal, non-local, faster than light transmissions would be necessary to satisfy the characteristics of phenomena in fifth dimensional, harmonic processes. This can not be experimentally demonstrated as yet, but the significance of these discoveries in the support they provide on an experimental level for an electrochemical-magnetic communications process which transcends duality and joins third and fifth dimensional actions in a biochemical, organismic, electromagnetic, psychophysiological field is encouraging.

The Principle of Action Potential

We are investigating the question of how memories may be recorded, stored, and transmitted in the context of a bi-dimensional system each operating under different rules, yet somehow remaining in extensive communication with each other.

In the problem of the particle-wave dilemma, scientists have been trying to find the answer to the question of how the photon in the interference experiment appears to know what to do, and to do it faster than the speed of light, shifting from particle to wave, throwing alternating light and dark lines on the screen instead of a circle of light, when the experimenter introduces two slits instead of just one to the photon. (See Chapter 7, "Quantum Physical Reality" for complete description.) The word "remembers" could easily be substituted for the word "knows". Therefore, at this juncture, the dilemma of how it "knows" whether to show up as a circle or lines can be viewed as rhetorical rather than actual. Atoms have experiences within their nuclei of protons and neutrons in relation to electrons which come and go. They have capabilities of response to events impinging upon them and those responses may be determined by more factors than we are able to scientifically pin down. The assumption we have to make, to make any sense of the particle-wave dilemma, is that inherent in the makeup of the atom is a capacity for responses to particle and wave bits of information with a potential for different responses to different stimuli. We don't yet know if that "memory" is in the particle or in the field which guides it.

The particle and the wave can be described as energy which changes its manifest form according to an action potential defined by the constraints presented in a particular environment. Atoms carry within them potentials for action - in this case to manifest in either a particle or a wave form, that is, to exist in a somewhat boundaried particle state or a less boundaried wave state. We have called the carrier of this energy with a potential for action a quonticle which travels within the electromagnetic environment of the quontic loop. A potential for action can have innumerable latent possibilities within itself and in that sense it can also constitute a memory bank in its own context. This memory for an action potential is a factor in the continuity and consistency inherent in the inanimate material as well as the organic universe. Does such memory, however, need to be a part of conscious memory any more than other quantum mechanical effects are a part of conscious memory? Memory on the level of quantum atomic activity is memory for an action potential. Memory on the level of genetic activity is also memory for an action potential. Physics memory and biological memory work within different environmental constraints so each of them contains its own specific framework of action potentials. Human memory, we must assume from the way life has evolved, contains both physics and biological memory at some level or we could not function at all. That just seems like common sense and doesn't need scientific proof. Therefore, the Freudian definition of memory in terms defining conscious and unconscious factors, valuable as it has been, is another constrained view of memory limited to and defined by its own peculiarly manifested framework of human behavior.

The "Map" — Memory Action Potential

The function of memory is to contain and transmit information when an opportunity for doing so presents itself. The transmission of its information may require a transformation in its form from one carrier to another type of carrier viz; from nerve impulse to verbal statement; more esoterically, from a fifth dimensional memory for an action potential into a third dimensional memory for an action potential.

If the energy of the photon or its field carries inherently all the information or memory available about one and two slits for all particles and waves, then it has no need for further information. All the possibilities exist, and are contained within the quantum of energy and its field for any action it might possibly take. This can be both a third and a fifth dimensional memory for action potential. However, on the three dimensional level of action potentials, one slit means that its potential for action is limited to the manifestation that we call a particle and two slits means that its potential for action is limited to the manifestation we call a wave within the constraints of action potentials accessible on planet Earth.

On another planet with different electromagnetic and biological structures the conditions under which the photon could manifest itself would be changed, therefore its response would shift accordingly. The particle-wave dilemma is the one particularly native to life on Earth and it is quite possible to conceive the presence of other environments which posit different kinds of limitations and possibilities than life on Earth. In each environment the energy which we see manifested in the particle wave dilemma finds which action is appropriate for which occasion. In our environment, the photon acts in the context of light waves and other electromagnetic phenomena which compose its earth-bound, quantum structure.

Indeed, it is known that electromagnetic waves from the earliest conditions of the universe such as the hypothetical Big Bang still exist and there are galaxies whose light waves, originating billions of years ago, are just now reaching the earth. Therefore there are "memories" of the earliest conditions in our universe which may just be manifesting themselves to us now, and other memories in the form of light waves are currently existing that will not manifest for many centuries to come.

It seems as if without memories chaos would reign without let-up. However, even chaos is seen in physics today as the source of much that is novel and creative rather than as something dysfunctional and destructive. If one doesn't fear chaos, change and creative action lead to welcome, sometimes awesome solutions. Underneath chaos it is recognized that an invisible layer of subtle organization exists which actually becomes evident through the unfolding and passage of chaotic events. In that sense, it might be said that the patterns that underlie chaos are reflections of a fifth-dimensional memory whose action potential becomes manifest in the third dimension first as chaos, secondly as pattern, thirdly as structure and finally as form. Looking at it this way, chaos may be interpreted as the first step in a transformation of energy states, part of the process of interchanges and transformations between fifth and third dimensions, rather than as a steady, unchangeable state.

To the casual observer, chaos looks like an unboundaried condition of total disorganization with unpredictable energies. However, chaos is found to take place within the context of a system that is inherently ongoing and subtly orderly (Barrow 1988). When the seemingly chaotic event is looked at on the quantum level it is seen to carry in it the seeds of a larger organized structure - in other words it has a subtly organized action potential. This process view of chaos is just as significant for human affairs as it is in the study of physics.

Resonance

How do the psychic and physical dimensions interact in the human being? Consciousness serves the bodymind as the physical projection screen on which events play out the psychological, physiological and psychic characteristics of a person's life. New experiments in bioenergetic systems are beginning to confirm that energy transfers both within and between physical and non-physical systems or, body and mind, that transcend the speed of light are indeed possible. In this type of transformation, the energy can be transmitted from the harmonic to the reality level even though a person, ostensibly, has not asked for it. The effective strength of accumulations of unconscious experience, perhaps including past lives, with or without direction from the conscious mind, may trigger a harmonic resonance, thereby intruding itself into conscious experience on the three dimensional reality plane. The extent and intensity with which an unconscious experience is transformed into conscious experience is due to the memory's action potential. That probably sounds like a lot of jargon so it will have to be explained.

An action potential is an electromagnetic energy field which is in a pre-transmission and therefore pre-transformation phase. Through the effects of resonance, the action potential can be transformed into an active electromagnetic energy field. A resonance is a joining together of separated electromagnetic fields. In this process we are talking about resonance between the three-dimensional and fifth dimensional levels communicating through the medium of the quonticle travelling in the quontic loop. Resonance, or tuning in, between the two dimensions may be increased in strength through the accumulation of conscious or unconscious experiences in the course of a person's lifetime. John Eccles, a neurologist who won a Nobel prize for his neurological discoveries, as well as other research neurologists, have been working on the idea of an electromagnetic "gate". Briefly, the level of accessibility through the gate depends on the accumulated neurobiological massing of electrochemical connections activated by the triggering consciousness (or unconscious energy) of the person. The gate is a concept that is applicable to three-dimensional consciousness.

However, we are proposing that memory and consciousness do not lie solely within the physiological body of a person. The physiological explanation appears inadequate for the complex phenomena of human experience.

New experiments such as the one quoted above in bioenergetic systems are beginning to confirm that psychophysiological energy transfers both within and between physical and non-physical systems that transcend the speed of light are indeed possible. The next chapter discusses the way this might occur. With faster than light transformation, it would be possible for energy to be transmitted from the harmonic to the reality level through the quontic loop even though a person, ostensibly, has not asked for it. Accumulations of unconscious experience builds the action potential on both the fifth and third dimensional levels through resonance experiences. This could conceivably include any paranormal experience from dejá vu to past lives.

A resonance is a joining together through reverberation and amplification of two vibrations whose frequency is the same, or nearly the same, as the natural vibrations of each. A common example is a glass breaking when an opera singer's voice reaches the right pitch, causing a sound vibration which is the same as the natural vibration of the glass. In our extended structure we are talking about resonance between the three-dimensional and fifth dimensional levels communicating through the medium of the quonticle in the quontic loop in which the form separating the two structures cracks due to their resonance, just as the glass does. It's as if their boundaries, in dissipating permit a kind of entropy to occur which allows the differences between the structures to mix together in some degree. Such an instance incurs a vibrational and resonance dynamic coming from each source which triggers a connection between the third and fifth dimensions allowing their energies to mix in the quontic loop.

The above statements are provocative, to say the least. They suggest ideas which may or may not ultimately be supported by further experimentation. It is supposed that persons who continually practice to learn and develop their transpersonal, spiritual, or psychic skills and capabilities internally will accumulate the same type of neuropsychological structures, opening gates, developing resonant vibrations for fifth dimensional memory and consciousness as they can and do for other phenomenological life events. In doing so they create and increase their access-ability to the quontic loop enabling them to reach into and draw upon psychic experiences as part of their daily lives.

(See Figure 22., *Model of Homeostatic Memory with Consciousness Feedback Loop*, a broad outline of the relationships between the psychophysiological and the psychic levels of existence and their interactions through feedback.)

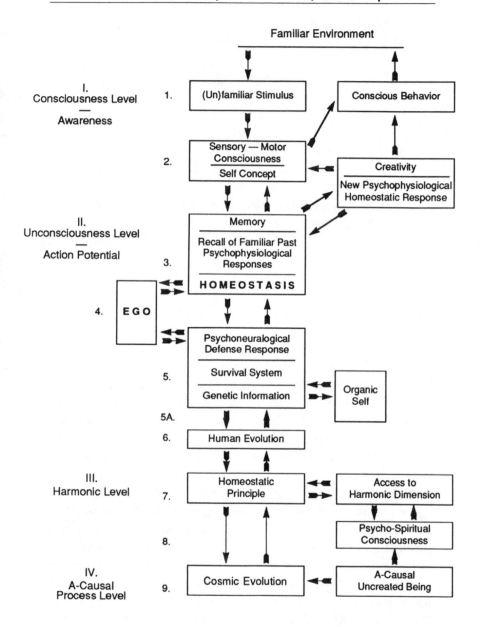

Figure 22.
Model of Homeostatic Memory
with Consciousness Feedback Loop

Non-Linear Light Waves: Photonics

> "For an idea that does not at first seem insane,
> there is no hope.
>
> — Albert Einstein

It's All Those Insane Relativities

I really like Albert Einstein. Coming from an empirical physicist the statement above may seem astounding, but he has the reputation for having built relativity on subjective or intuitive processes and mathematical reasoning, with objective proof of his ideas coming later. He had a truly unifunctional mind.

The question we are asking now is whether relativity theory has any relationship to homeostasis and the fifth dimension in quontic psychology; and the question may indeed seem insane. Sometimes, "insane" simply means that the rational mind has difficulty comprehending the logical connections between the parts of thoughts, but if such connections can be demonstrated then the idea can be given rational consideration and evaluated for its possible sanity. Even Relativity received condemnation when it first appeared. It contained ideas that could not at first be verified and connected with the real world because it required a break with Newtonian physics.

In essence then, what does relativity have to say about paranormal experience, and about past lives in particular?

Some review of relativity is first necessary. It has two basic postulates. Briefly, let's review its basic ideas again.

1. Motion and the perception of speed is not absolute. They are relative to the framework of the perceiver.

2. The speed of light is a universal constant at 186,000 miles per second.

What does that mean in terms of practical experience?

For the first one, suppose you are in a stationary train opposite another train in a railroad station. Suddenly you perceive the other train moving out of the station. This continues until you observe a post on the platform that seems to be moving backwards and you immediately realize that you are on the moving train and the other one is standing still. You needed the third frame of reference given you by the post, which experience has told you is incapable of independent movement, to perceive that you were indeed on the moving object. An object moving in free space will not perceive its own movement and will perceive motion in the objective frame of reference. However, there is no such thing as "objective" movement. Perception of motion is not absolute and is relative to the frame of reference seen by the perceiver. In other words, either train could be seen as moving, and it doesn't matter which.

The second postulate seems clear enough, but it too requires a new way of looking at things. In a three dimensional framework, if a car going 50 mph overtakes a bike going 10 mph, the perceived difference between their speeds from the biker's point of view is 40 mph. In a relativity framework, space and time are joined in the fourth dimension. This means space and time define one another; you can't measure space without time (miles per hour) and can't measure time without an equivalent space within which it occurs. Therefore, distances between stars and galaxies are measured in light-years; the amount of time is equivalent to the amount of space between objects. Time and space are equally important to each other's definition and join to become the fourth dimension.

In this framework, the speed of light being a constant means that it is not affected by three dimensional space and time measurements and remains the same under all circumstances. Thus, if you are in a spaceship going 185,000 mps and a photon passes by your window will you see it going 1 mph, consistent with the third dimensional situation? Not so. In relativity, constancy means that the photon is going 186,000 mps faster than your speed of 185,000 mps. Does that mean it is going 371,000 mps? No, that can't be either since its speed is a universal constant. Lightspeed is 186,000 mps constantly and is not relative to the frame of reference of any other object.

The speed of light has other consequences which, expressed in three-dimensional terms, make no sense and look absolutely insane. In the course of accelleration toward lightspeed the following would be observed taking place:

1. Clocks slow down to become zero at lightspeed
  .
2. Distances, length, becomes shorter, reaching zero at lightspeed.

3. Mass increases to reach infinity at lightspeed.

Actually, these effects are present at all times at any speed, but at the slow movements occurring on Earth none of these effects are visible. There is the well-known conundrum of the twins born at the same time, one of which lives in a fast moving space-ship in outer space, the other living on Earth, meeting 60 years later. The Earthling is 60 years of age while the space inhabitant is literally only 30 years of age. All movement, even organic clocks slow down when accelerating toward lightspeed.

To further break down the meaning of the effects of the

speed of light let us suppose that Allen is in a spacecraft accelerating toward the speed of light while being observed by Becky who is travelling at a constant speed or is at rest.

a. Becky will observe Allen's clock to be slowing down relative to hers. The length of Allen's spacecraft, indeed Allen himself will be perceived to grow shorter while she and hers remain the same; and at the same time both Allen and his spacecraft will increase in mass as they accellerate, while hers remains the same.

b. The effects happening to Allen as pereceived from Becky's framework are identical to the effects perceived by Allen happening to Becky from within his framework. He does not perceive himself and his spacecraft moving, but perceives Becky and her spacecraft to be the one accelerating toward the speed of light. No wonder men and women have such unresolvable misunderstandings. (See Figure 23., *Allen and Becky — Who's Accelerating? A little misunderstanding.*)

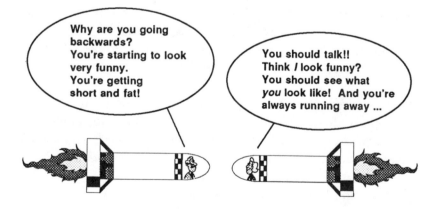

Figure 23.
Allen and Becky — Who's Accellerating?
A little misunderstanding.

To these standard effects of the speed of light I would like to add the following observations:

c. At maximum lightspeed these effects become zero or infinite. Thus a condition of timelessness, dimensionlessness and masslessness develops. Zero time, zero space and infinite mass -none of which is measureable and therefore equal zero - coexist at lightspeed. Since zero and infinite states cannot be measured they cannot be described in three-dimensions. We cannot see what goes on in a relativistic perspective at or past the speed of light even though we may theorize and have intuition about it.

d. Observation "c" is also the condition of the quontic psychological fifth dimension pertaining beyond the barrier of the fourth dimension, that is, beyond the barrier of lightspeed. This is also presumably the "spacetime" from which all paranormal phenomena originate before they manifestly occur in three-dimensional spacetime.

e. Consciousness therefore also has the appearance of a duality, having a three-dimensional, practical frame of reference in time and space and a fifth-dimensional unmeasureable frame of reference which is even beyond measurement in relativity, simultaneously.

Perceived from Earth, sunlight takes eight minutes to arrive from the sun, but perceived from the point of view of the speed of light which has zero space, time and mass, it leaves the sun and arrives on the Earth simultaneously, travelling no distance in no time.

How can this be? No one has explained it, it just is. It is our metaphor for consciousness. Consciousness appears to take time to happen in the course of events on earth, but its source is fifth-dimensional where neither time, space or mass exist. Although, in earth terms it is fragmented, it manifests the essence of a unifunctional operational mode, needing no time for its presence to appear, having the capability of simultaneity or synchronicity (Jung 1983). These dualities pervade quantum physics as well as relativity and appear to be a fundamental condition of the way the universe functions. It is not simply a rejectable "new age" point of view, it is fundamental to science. That being the case, it must apply to human as well as non-human functioning, and we propose that the human vehicle for dual states is consciousness.

Further Implications

There are further implications that can be drawn up as hypotheses from the observations offered above:

1. All the divisions beteen subjective vs. objective, material vs. mental, three-dimensional vs. five-dimensional, mind vs. body, are arguments without any substance. None of these categories have an independent temporal or spacial existence. There is a mutual delusion on the part of practitioners of Science and Mysticism, Eastern and Western Philosophies, because matter doesn't come from mind, or consciousness, any more than mind is a product of physical matter, or the brain. They exist together, that is, they coexist in a unifunctional reality, like Allen and Becky, in a state of co-dependency, each perceiving the faults of the other without realizing those faults could not even be perceived, no less denied into non-existence, without their co-dependent condition.

Co-dependency has become a dirty word in psychotherapy and it may be relative in strength in interpersonal relations, but may never be denied completely as an ultimate quality of relationship. Each of them exist only within the framework of the other's existence as elements in a process of interactions.

2. Subjective and objective reality are ultimately, in the absolute sense, unknowable. They don't exist as independent

frames of reference and are therefore unknowable except from the framework of the other. That framework is defined by the relativistic interactions that occur between them. There is no such thing is "subjective truth" or "objective truth" except in relation to the truth of the other and the rules of relativistic interactions that pertain to their joint frame of reference.

3. The above is a condition of human as well as non-human existence since it is the framework of conditions for all existence as far as can be ascertained. The relativistic interactions that occur among events based on the codependency between all phenomena is another way of describing the framework of operations under which the Homeostatic Principle also exists.

Perception of Past Lives from a Relativistic Framework

Since Becky and Allen see the clocks of the other slowing down while theirs continues at a regular rate, the clock in the other frame appears to be going backward in time. Therefore, in the receiver's frame, a message sent from one ship to the other is sent at a time that is the future of the receiver, but is perceived by the sender as a message received in the distant past of the receiver.

In absolute time, which does not exist, the messages may have been sent and received within moments of each other, but that is not possible unless both ships were travelling at identical speeds. Changes in space affect changes in time so any slowing down in speed would affect times as well as distances. Perception of past events occurring in the course of present events and perception of future events in the course of present events are a necessity in a relativistic framework.

The Insane Consequences of Relativity for Consciousness

What takes time to travel from place to place, yet can be in two places simultaneously? What can be a particle or a wave, is massless and has no definitive shape or form of its own, yet has been instrumental in creating the Earth's physical environment? Only light can fulfill that description, unless you call it God.

A model for consciousness? It's also a model for the force of gravity. Massless, no shape or form of its own, not a thing, yet affecting the actions of forms and masses. In three dimensions it seems to need time to travel from place to place, yet it also appears to be everywhere simultaneously. It determines the principles of interactions for a major part of life on earth. It seems to engage in universal and specific, or non-linear and linear modes of interaction simultaneously.

In consciousness, thoughts generate specific actions but the source of thoughts seems hard to locate specifically. Thought is an outcome of consciousness, like the flow of water is an outcome of turning on the faucet. It always seems to be available from its own reservoir without having to be put there. Consciousness, like light, seems to have no beginning and no end, as if it were the outcome of a principle rather than a three-dimensional, empirical, living and dying beginning and ending. Yet they both can interact and have profound effects upon things that do have empirical beginnings and endings.

Light and consciousness have a constancy of their own. Light always travels 186,000 mps faster than anything in its environment so there is no beginning speed and there is no ending speed. It begins and ends at the identical speed, yet itself needs no speed whatsoever. Space follows the same rules as time, therefore seems intricately bound up with light. We've already seen how it helps to form consciousness.

Without linear space the effects of light would not be evident to us any more than the effects of time and motion would be evident to us. There appears to be a co-dependent triumvirate in the manifestation and actions of what we call space, time and light. Neither would the effects of consciousness be apparent without the presence of that triumvirate. Are they a mutually co-dependent foursome?

I suspect there is a fifth member that belongs to this group and it is Gravity. Space, time, light, and gravity as scientifically studied objects would seem not to need consciousness, but according to metaphysical beliefs they are manifestations of consciousness and are dependent on it. Are they all like heads and tails, various ways of describing the same events? What they have in common is the difficulty in discerning beginnings and endings, a lack of diminution and increase in their quantities or their qualities until placed in the form of an object that can be empirically manipulated.

Consciousness perceives three-dimensional reality in a certain way but the Copenhagen interpretation points out that that is relativistic. The reality of the operation of consciousness doesn't become manifest until consciousness has done something to reality. And without the reality of three-dimensional objects and events we would not be aware of consciousness. Consciousness and reality external to it co-create each other. They are equal parts of Reality. For a representation of this situation see Figure 24., Matrix One, the incorporation of knowledge regarding four major forms of energy-stuff in physics with that of psychology, interacting and co-creating each other.

The Seen is the Seer

As Alfred North Whitehead stated, "What is seen and the one who sees it are identical, the seer is the seen and the seen is the seer". That follows squarely out of relativity. The seer and the seen are one in their mirror image as well as in their delusions. That also means there is no objective or subjective reality except in terms of seen and seer.

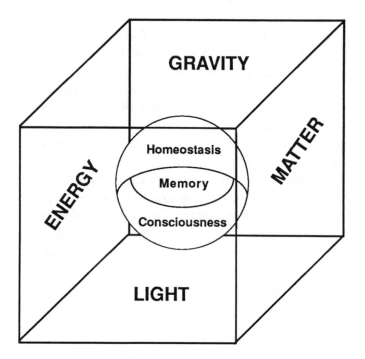

Figure 24.
Matrix One,

the incorporation of knowledge regarding four major forms of energy-stuff in physics with that of psychology, interacting and co-creating each other.

Data is the outcome of a relativistic process of interaction between subject and object. Objectivity and subjectivity aren't real independently because their data can only be the manifestation of the availability of a relativistic, unifunctional process of interaction. Consciousness, which is known only subjectively, doesn't and can't actually know itself as a purely subjective phenomenon. It can only know itself vis a vis a relationship with an object, or through memories of such relationships. It follows, therefore, that anyone who thinks he knows the total truth about himself or about an object in absolute terms is deluding himself, if not altogether crazy.

If nothing else, understanding the relativity of knowledge accessible from either consciousness or objective data should make us feel humble. The limitations we have to deal with as well as the amount of knowledge ultimately available are equally awesome.

However, the Homeostatic Principle maintains a balance between objective and subjective inputs into a reality framework. It allows for the three-dimensional delusional aspect of perception and makes the necessary corrections to keep within a relativistic frame of reference. In other words, the only way to keep a balance in things is to allow for a certain amount of delusion in your perceptions and in your relationships, so you can allow the swing in your homeostatic pendulum to happen. Any description of the totality of reality must include delusional as well as corrective perceptions.

The source of the Homeostatic Principle is fifth dimensional and therefore it functions within the rules of the quontic field which is oneness among events. It becomes three dimensional and maintains the unifunctional mind as its orientation within three dimensional reality, thus supporting survival and homeostasis in that framework. Quontic Psychology thus manages to include both levels of operations simultaneously while explaining how they are connected.

Complementarism —
Particle and Wave Revisited:
Healing the Splits

Einstein's statement that 'God does not play dice with the universe', a witty rebuttal to the quantum physical principle of uncertainty, stimulated Neils Bohr to reply, 'In my impudent way I would say that ...no one - not even the dear Lord himself - can know what an expression like throwing dice means.'

— Pais - Niels Bohr's Times [1]

A Clash of Genius

Well, now, looking at that controversy externally from the metaphysical point of view the question is who has the better knowledge of how the dear Lord behaves? It was a wonderful controversy that lasted over many years, beginning in 1927 and continuing into the 1930's that made both men sharpen their ideas as well as the minds of those around them about quantum physics. However, it didn't resolve anything about the dice throwing inclinations of the Lord. The metaphysical position might be that since God is Lord of the Unseen Universe he is ultimately unknowable in his deepest recesses. Today's truth leans toward Bohr because we may never know whether God knows about or engages in crap shoots; we can only pick at miserly clues because the inclination of the Lord for self-revelation is frustratingly negligible.

The issues of the controversy were vital to each of these immense geniuses. It was based on Bohr's support for quantum physics as a probabilistic science in which nature's knowable parts and processes were subject to the principle of uncertainty and an experimenter's design in setting up his research, while Einstein believed in the irrevocable existence of an objectively given universe. Both of these men's positions were rooted in the manner of interpreting the particle-wave dilemma; the Copenhagen interpretation of course coming out of the research work of Bohr and his associates, including Heisenberg, and the challenge to it coming mainly from Einstein - following his great contributions.

Bohr contributed, among many important ideas, the central idea of complementarity in response to the question of the particle-wave dilemma. Complementarity developed in Bohr's thinking as a way to accept the mounds of evidence built up experimentally in support of the fact that the electron, as well as the proton, could manifest in the form of either a wave or as a particle. The complementarity principle states that neither form of observation is incorrect, that each is in some aspect complementary and therefore necessary to the other.

It followed from Heisenberg's demonstration in early 1927 that it was not possible to determine accurately both the momentum and the position of a particle simultaneously. The more accurately one was measured, the less accurate the other became. Thus the principle of uncertainty, which was also decribed earlier in the quantum physics chapter, provided a mathematical way of handling this dilemma so that it began to function by providing further information to researchers.

Bohr was more of a philosopher than Heisenberg and realized that there was a more general principle at work in the particle-wave duality. He sought to get underneath the duality of the particle whereas Heisenberg believed that all of nature existed primarily in the context of the mathematical explanation. Bohr was also unwilling to discard classical explanation altogether in quantum physics believing that the classical must always precede the quantum explanation in a continuous way, calling this relationship the correspondence principle. Even though formal Newtonian and quantum mathematics differed in the microcosm, on the macrocosmic scale they merged into a collaborative explanation. Heisenberg was determined in saying there was a point where the application of classical theory ended and quantum theory began. That was how he saw his uncertainty principle, as another domain of function in the universe. He stated,

> "When we get beyond this range of the classical theory, we must realize that our words don't fit. They don't really get a hold on the physical reality and therefore a new mathematical scheme is just as good as anything because the new mathematical scheme then tells what may be there and what may not be there. Nature just in some way follows the scheme".

"We must realize that our words don't fit" will ring a bell with every metaphysical researcher. The world of quantum behavior is no longer the same, it does not follow the same rules as mass, energy, momentum, etc. in classical physics. That was what made it so hard to articulate both mathematically and verbally the dilemma of the particle wave duality, followed by many additional hard to resolve if not unresolvable problems, such as the Bohr-Einstein conflict regarding the nature of reality noted at the beginning of this chapter.

One of the major unresolved effects of the uncertainty principle (and perhaps the one that perturbed Einstein the most) is that it unseats the classical notions of causality. Newtonian physics states that if precise initial position and momentum of a particle are provided then exact prediction of position and velocity can be made at a future time. Not so in quantum mechanics in which exact conditions of both position and momentum can never be provided, therefore the predication of future on past behavior is not possible. Causality just doesn't work at the quantum level, but uncertainty and probability do. Thus, Einstein's protest about the image of God playing dice.

Heisenberg came out with his uncertainty paper in early 1927 and Bohr with his complementarity paper in late 1927. The essential thrust of Bohr's argument was that although a wave and a particle are mutually exclusive at the times that they manifest themselves to an observer they are both fundamental and necessary to the understanding of the object's properties.

The differences between these two men's positions can be seen to have acquired another focus in the context of this book. The idea of the quantum leap in the transformation of the wave into the particle is similar to Heisenberg's way of seeing classical and quantum worlds as being discrete and discontinuous. The idea of there being a quantum loop which contains the functions of the conversion process from wave to particle in a form that is continuous is similar to Bohr's principles of correspondence and complementarity. Even though there are rules of operation in each (wave and particle) which are peculiar and inseparable from the mode of functioning in each domain, there is a communication process between them which affords continuity. This is just as true in human affairs between the mundane and the quontic reality experience as it is in physics between the Newtonian and quantum reality experience.

In the quontic domain the problem that arises is also similar to the early problems in the quantum domain. How do you describe and explicate functions and operations of phenomena happening in a domain for which language, up that point, does not exist with a language that does exist? "We are suspended in language", said Bohr. There repeatedly comes that point where "our words don't fit", said Heisenberg.

They were both right. We must have new words and a new model, which is what the quantum theorists provided for physics, and as we have attempted to provide in this book.

The Range of Complementarity

The mistake of the quantum physicist theoreticians has been to believe that physics offers all the answers to the human experience of life on earth, whereas by the very nature of its frame of investigation and discourse it is impossible for physics to do that. It is easy to agree that research in physics has led it into areas which are probably vital to those in the human experience, but differences between physics and psychology are just as important as their similarities.

Physicists, obviously, are not committed to researching the dynamics of human experience on either a daily or a universal, cosmic basis. The human experience requires a uniquely human understanding, which is what the quontic psychological model provides. However, physical and psychological models, though worlds apart in many ways, also manifest a complementariness. Obviously, in human experience, the psychological world does not exist without a physical world for its context and the physical world does not exist without a psychological world for its context. Each only gains reality through the presence of the other, which is the significance of complementariness. That is the same thought that I presented in Figure 2., in which I demonstrated that the spiritual/metaphysical and mundane/scientific explanations of reality were incomplete and fragmented without the other. With complementarity we have come full circle.

Bohr did not think that his principle of complementarity was exclusively limited to physics. Perhaps only intuitively, he was the first physicist to think about the way other sciences might benefit from the application of the complementarity concept and therefore was the first to demonstrate the FOCUS viewpoint. In particular he spoke about "complementarism" (as Pais P. 439 calls it) in Psychology, Human Cultures, Biology and Epistemology. Since our major concern is the psychological aspect in such relationships, I will not recount what he says about the others.

Complementarism shows up in psychology in several different ways, according to Bohr. There is the complementary nature of subject and object. The subject is the perceiver of the thing being perceived which is the object. The distinction between subject and object becomes something of an illusion since neither can be said to exist without the presence of the other.

He also suggests that life, which is inseparably connected with consciousness and death have a similar complementariness. This is only briefly mentioned in Pais, but to expand that thought, it can be added that we know about death only because we have consciousness about life, and we accept that life for some reason needs to end in death, which is also the end of consciousness, at least in its material aspect. Consciousness might continue in another perhaps more essential form after death but we don't know whether the reverse is also true, that is, that death needs to end in life, either on the immaterial or the material planes, though many say that it does, at least in the sense of completing one's Karmic potentials. The doubting person would not regard life and death capable of engaging in true complementary relationships whereas the person believing in Karma and "life after death" would. They would see life and death as well as consciousness on a functional continuum, separation provided only by the forms of their manifestation.

Actor and spectator are another set of complementary relationships, in Bohr's thinking. Being a spectator provides the reflective, evaluative role for the person who then will leave that role to become the actor. During action he does not engage in the spectator role so that the two become mutually exclusive even though they are both basic elements in a person's mental content (namely, they are both necessary in consciousness). While in a spectator and reflecting state one cannot act and while in a state of complete action one cannot reflect.

I would add that the latter is not necessarily completely true in that one's actions may provide an immediate feedback into reflection which can then halt or change the action. Reflection by the same token can lead into some immediate action, so again we can see that there is a powerful and continuous relationship between them despite the mutually exclusive modality in which they express themselves.

He sets up a more complicated relationship between "the state of consciousness in the description of which words like *I will* find application...[and its] complementary...state in which we are concerned with an analysis of motives for our actions" (Pais, P.440). Bohr associates the analysis of motivation to reasoning which, in its turn, is complementary to the subjective emotional state of feeling freedom. Becoming engaged in actions of will, one has a feeling of freedom and renounces reasoning with explanations, (at least for the time being).

This leads directly into the most conventional complementariness in the relationship between thoughts and feelings. (There isn't further description of Bohr's ideas about this in Pais, so what follows is my own elaboration). The conventional attitude about thoughts and feelings, or emotions, is that they are mutually exclusive, that one is either a thinking person or a feeling person, and that one may be thinking about another person or about an event without having feeling about it.

However, in this very conventional case I don't think the analogy completely holds up very well in terms of contemporary psychology. It is understood that there may be a severe conflict between thinking and emotions with thought, reasoning, and reflection being used to control and dissipate emotions while, if one behaves emotionally there is no possibility of thinking.

In their extremes it cannot be denied that this is probably the mode of operation. But that would not be the healthiest manifestation of consciousness. An ideal state would be one in which feelings and thoughts behave in a collaboration in which a person would be having feeling even while thinking about something and would have perspective enough to reflect even in the course of feeling about something. Perhaps the strength of the emotions involved would be a key to determining whether modifcations from thought would be available during an emotional state. It might be said then that there is a complementariness between thought and emotions in which they can react either with mutual exclusion or may have an intrinsically supportive dialogue.

The Tao of Complementarism

Their similarity is too obvious not to compare Yin and Yang with Bohr's complementarism and correspondence principle. Bohr, like Freud, rejected all implications he might ever have engaged in metaphysical thinking, though he allowed that he permitted himself to philosophize, even to psychologize. This comment does not downgrade the value of Bohr's wider application of the principle of complementarity. If anything, it intends to point out that the applications of it are even wider than he would have allowed himself to see in that it does extend into the idea of the Tao that there is continuity in all things, even into things in the unseen universe which are impalpable to the senses.

Eastern mysticism has it that the complementary nature of material and immaterial reality are such that in order to fully grasp the experience of the unseen universe one must condition oneself to renounce all sensorially satisfying and ego gratifying objects. Such a "death" of the operations of the material self while still engaging in a process of living is not easy to attain, but it points up the acceptance of the mutually exclusive nature of mystic experience in the case of the most practiced yogis.

We don't aspire to such a fulfillment of the mutually exclusive possibilities inherent in complimentariness in daily life. We look more toward that aspect of it that permits the flow of relationships instead of the mutually exclusive aspects of a state. It is the Yin and Yang of continuity between the opposites that engages us in working out the contradictions that normally provoke how we behave. It is valuable to know that those contradictions are not something to be buried in fear and guilt but that they can be assumed to be the way the material universe functions normally, even in physics.

Complementariness and the correspondence principle also offers us some of the best evidence that physics can offer regarding the universal operation of the underlying principle of homeostasis. The opposition of the quantum to the Newtonian is more illusory than real since one cannot exist without the other. The contradictions between Bell's a-causal, a-temporal hidden universe and the Newtonian causal, temporal universe are also due here more to Maya than matter. They exist in a field of mutually interdependent interactions: a feedback condition of the homeostatic principle operating toward the fulfillment of the survival of its objects, with a rope of dependency connecting them and their functions, nurtured by the homeostatic principle.

We have repeatedly pointed out that the only way that these relationships could remain in balance is through the principle of homeostasis. It allows the flow between the ends of the continuum to remain connected, offering guidance through feedback keeping individuals, societies and even the universe in some sort of survival condition. It is the prerequisite for all the rest.

Finally, I would like to point out that the vast undertakings of scientific research and practice are themselves a product of the homeostatic principle. Keeping in mind that homeostasis takes place in the service of survival with memory and feedback as its major first-line assistants, it is impossible to think of any significant scientific work fulfilling its goals without the essential utilization of these four components of our paradigm.

Science's major value by its own definition, whether in physics, medicine, chemistry, biology, etc. is to augment the body of information available, gathering knowledge which will secure our place in the universe against the unpredictable and often destructive forces of nature. Nature can be very destructive to man's survival through its weather conditions, attacks on the physical survival of the body, as well as through mankind's attacks on himself and his own kind. This leads us very often unfortuntately into the catch-22 of killing the subject while intending to cure the disease. We've pointed this out in the case of the use of medical cures employing drugs as overkill (Miller 1993) and now we have it again in the case of nuclear energy.

Nevertheless, the good news is that we will not destroy the universe, we will not even destroy the earth with such tools of survival as the hydrogen bomb and civilian comforts as nuclear reactors. We can destroy ourselves, but homeostasis is much bigger than we are. We live in complementariness, in the loop of chaos and harmony. It will go on, take the measure of the Yin-Yang of it and with Lao Tse's helping wisdom nature will make the necessary corrections for the state of imbalance which we created as earth's creatures. Then, a new cosmic organic, homeostatic process will establish a new set of forces with a new set of creatures that, following their evolutionary developmental action potentials, will fulfill a new optimum way of functioning within its environment, to survive until the next particle-wave dilemma arrives. Hopefully. before making a new set of evolutionary creatures necessary, we'll solve it better than we have up to now.

To return to the opening quotations for this chapter, I don't knowwhether God plays dice with the universe, but we, the human race, certainly are doing that with our lives. And we do know what dice are and are aware of its statistics, so we can't blame God.

On the next page, we arrive at *A Plan for the Twenty-First Century*, which offers some ideas about how to return ourselves and our Earth to a homeostatic environment.

A Plan for the Twenty-First Century

1. Healing Culture and Society Through FOCUS

The development of science as a unifunctional process of study. The overall integration of the three-dimensional sciences - whether physical, biological, or psychological - with their fifth dimensional counterparts in studies such as meta-physics and parapsychology. Ultimately incorporating the integration of body, mind, feeling and spirit within FOCUS.

2. Healing the Individual

Unification of medicine and alternative healing practices into a unifunctional diagnostic and treatment process. Make apt use of the tremendous diversity of healing possibilities beyond the limitations of medication. Affirm the primary involvement of the patient for a successful healing outcome. Offer patients available information regarding choices to make self-motivating decisions.

a. Empower people to accept themselves, their real feelings, their intuitions about themselves and others and to give up repression as a way of life. Affirm that contact with feelings means contact with the body as a place where love, pleasure, sensitivity, and respect for the feelings and bodies of others is primary.

b. Empower, contact and forward development of the spiritual self. The Homeostatic Principle is fully able to operate on the human dimension when the above are the basic values input through the unifunctional process.

3. Healing the Planet

Establish Gaia as a responsible view of how homeostasis operates on Earth. Restoration of the American Indian philosophy of collaboration with nature as a way of life, instigation of industrial changes to implement the above values. Outlawing war and weapons as an option for individuals and nations to solve their differences. Move from the stuck point of weapons and warfare into a larger view of homeostasis.

References

Introduction and Overview

1. Woolger, Roger. (1985) Other Lives, Other Selves. N.Y.: Doubleday.

2. Perls, Fritz. (1969) Gestalt Therapy Verbatim. CA.: Real People Press.

3. Janov, Arthur. (1970) The Primal Scream. N.Y.: Dell.

4. Miller, Daniel. "Birth, Death and Organic Energy, Part One", Primal Community. Spring 1977. N.Y.: International Primal Accociation.

5. Miller, Daniel. "Birth, Death and Organic Energy, Part Two", Primal Community. Spring 1978. N.Y.: International Primal Accociation.

Chapter One

1. Clark, Ronald W. Einstein, The Life and Times. (1971) New York: Avon Books.

2. Ibid.

3. Lloyd, Seth. "The Calculus of Intricacy". The Sciences Sept.- Oct. 1990. Pp. 38-44.

4. Weber, R. (1982) "The Tao of Physics Revisited" in K. Wilber, Ed. The Holographic Paradigm P. 241. Boston: New Science Library, Shambala Press.

5. Pagels, H.R. (1987) "Complexity, A New Synthesis of the Sciences", an Executive Director's letter in Science Focus. New York: N.Y. Academy of Sciences, V.2, #2.

6. Weber, R. (1982). "What the Fuss is All About". Ch.3, P. 27-34 in K.Wilber, Ed. The Holographic Paradigm. Boston: Shambala Press.

7. Feynman, Richard. (1990). The Character of Physical Law. Cambridge, Mass: The M.I.T. Press. P.124-125.

Chapter Three

1. Blofield, John. (1980). Gateway to Wisdom. London:George Allen & Unwin, Ltd. P. 181.

2. John, Roy E. (1976) Models of Consciousness in Consciousness and Self-Regulation, Eds. Schwartz, D.E. and Shapiro, D., New York: Plenum.

3. St. John, Patricia. (1991) The Secret Language of the Dolphins. N.Y.: Summit Books.

4. Nozaki Yoshiyuki. Introduction to Buddhist Study. The Seikyo Times. World Tribune Press: Nichiren Shoshu of America. May, 1984.

5. Freud, Sigmund. (1943). A General Introduction To Psychoanalysis. New York: Garden City Publishing Co.

6. Jung, Carl. (1964). Man and His Symbols. New York:Dell
    Publishing Co.

7. Wambach, Helen. (1984) Reliving Past Lives. N.Y.:
    Barnes & Noble.

8. Stevenson, Ian. (1974) Twenty Cases Suggestive of Re-
    incarnation. Charlottesville: University Press of Virginia.

9. Andrade, Hernani Guimaraes. (1980). A Case Suggestive
    of Reincarnation: Jacira & Ronaldo. Monograph #3 of The
    Brazilian Institute for Psychobiophysical Research. Sao
    Paolo, Brazil.

Chapter Four

1. Pert, Candace B. "The Wisdom of the Receptors". Ad-
    vances . Publication of the Institute for the Advancement
    of Health. 3:3. Summer 1986:12.

2. Chamberlain, David B. "The Expanding Boundaries of
    Memory". Revision. Spring 1990. P. 16.

3. Ezzell, Carol. "Memories Might Be Made of This". Science
    News. May 25, 1991. V. 139, #21. P. 328-330.

4. Miller, Daniel. "The Psychobiological Nature of Reality
    with a Theory About Alzheimer's". Advances. Winter
    1992.

5. Jung, Carl. (1973) Synchronicity. N.J.: Princeton U.
    Press.

6. Jaynes, Julian (1976) The Origins of Consciousness in
    the Breakdown of the Bicameral Mind. Boston: Houghton
    Mifflin Co.

7. Pinchot, Roy B. Ed., 1984. The Brain. P. 92. N.Y.: Torstar.

8. Grof, Stanislov. (1985) Beyond the Brain. N.Y.: State University of New York Press.

9. Knutson, Peter. "Painter of Neurons" (on Santiago Ramon y Cajals) Science 85. Sept.

10. Johnson, George. "Scientists Identify 'Gate' in Brain as Crucial to Memory" in the N.Y. Times, Science Times section, May 10, 1988., Pp.C1 & C11.

11. Winson, Jonathan. "The Meaning of Dreams". Scientific American. Nov. 1990. P. 86-96.

Chapter Five

1. Cipra, Barry. "If You Can't See It, Don't Believe It" Science V.259 Jan. 1993, P.26-27.

2. Eccles, Sir John and Robinson, Daniel N. (1985) The Wonder of Being Human. Boston: Shambhala.

3. Gamow, George. (1958) Matter, Earth and Sky. Englewood Cliffs, N.J.: Prentice-Hall.

4. Herbert, Nick. (1985) Quantum Reality. New York: Penguin.

5. Von Neumann, J. (1955) Mathematical Foundations of Quantum Mechanics. Princeton University Press, Princeton, N.J.

6. Combs, A. and Holland, M. "Synchronicity in the House of Physics". Mindfield. Winter 1992, P.65-104.

Chapter Seven

1. Feynman, Richard P. and Weinberg, Steven. (1987). El-
    ementary Particles and the Laws of Physics. N.Y.: Cam-
    bridge U.

2. Pais, Abraham. (1991) Neils Bohr's Times.. Oxford, Eng:
    Clarendon Press.

3. Gamow, George. (1958) Matter, Earth and Sky. New
    York: Prentice-Hall. (P.291)

4. Talbot, Michael. (1988) Beyond the Quantum. New York:
    Doubleday. Bantam. P.24.

5. Einstein, A., Podolsky, B., and Rosen, N. (1935) Physics
    Review. 47, 777.

6. Sonea, Sorin. "The Global Organism". The Sciences. July,
    Aug. '88. Pp. 38-45.

7. Gribbin, John. (1984) In Search of Schrodinger's Cat.
    New York: Bantam.

8. Novick, Aaron and Cowley, Geoffrey. "An Imagined World".
    Book Review, Mind From Matter by Max Delbruck; ed-
    ited by Gunther S. Stent et al. Blackwell Scientific Pub-
    lications. The Sciences. N.Y. Academy of Sciences. Nov./
    Dec. 1986.

9. "Oscillating Chemical Waves Process Images", Science
    News, Feb. 11, 1989, Vol. 135. No. 6, P. 94.

10. Herbert, N. (1985) Quantum Reality: Beyond the New
    Physics. New York: Anchor Books, Doubleday. P. 115.

11. Pais, A. (1991) ... P. 235.

12. Pais, A. (1991)...P. 236.

13. Before having read the above in Pais, I'd conceived of the fifth dimensional domain which obviously has antecedents in other theories. What is satisfying is that I didn't realize there already was a theory proposed by a scientist of Bohr's stature that had come from quantum physics with similar qualities, thus suggesting reinforcement of quontic psychology's interactive and interconnective mind-matter model.

Chapter Eight

1. Von Baeyer, Hans Christian. The Sciences. "Dead Ringer". July/Aug. 1990. P. 2-4.

2. Clark, Ronald W. (1971) Einstein: The Life and Times. New York: World Publishing.

3. Becker, Robert O. (1985) The Body Electric: Electromagnetism and the Foundation of Life. New York: Morrow & Co.

4. Gerber, Richard (1988) Vibrational Medicine: New Choices for Healing Ourselves Santa Fe, N.M.: Bear & Co.

5. Redner, Briner & Snellman. "The Effects of a Bioenergetic Healing Technique on Chronic Pain". Subtle Energies. 1991, 2:3.

6. Ezzell, Carol. "Power-Line Static". Science News. Sept. 28, 1991, Vol. 140, NO. 13. P. 202-203.

7. Crease, & Mann. (1986). The Second Creation. New York:Macmillan Publishing Co. p.83.

8. Imry, Joseph and Webb, Richard A. "Quantum Interference and the Aharanov-Bohem Effect". Scientific American. Apr. 1989,   P. 56-62.

9. Ruthen, Russell. "Out of Its Field". Scientific American. Science and the Citizen, Oct. 1989. P. 26.

10. Feynman, Richard. (1985) Surely, You're Joking Mr. Feynman. New York: Norton.

11. Georgi, H.M. (1989) "Effective Quantum Field Theories" in Davies, Paul. The New Physics (P. 449) N.Y.: Cambridge U. Press.

Chapter Nine

1. Bell, J.S. (1987) Speakable and Unspeakable in Quantum Mechanics. N.Y. Cambridge University Press.

Chapter Ten

1. Lao Tsu Tao Te Ching A New Translation by Gia-Fu Feng and Jane English (New York: Random House. Vintage Books. 1972).

2. Prigogine, I. (1984) Order Out of Chaos N.Y: Bantam.

3. Thomsen, D.E. (1987) "In the Beginning was Quantum Mechanics". Science News. May 30. P.346.

4. Eccles, Sir John and Robinson, Daniel N. (1985). The Wonder of Being Human. Boston: Shambhala.

5. Hawking, Stephan. (1988) A Brief History of Time. New York: Bantam Doubleday Dell.

6. Petersen, Ivars. "A Different Dimension". Science News. May 27, 1989. P.328-330.

7. Bell, J.S. (1987) Speakable and Unspeakable in Quantum Mechanics. New York: Cambridge University Press. P. 94-96.

Chapter Twelve

1. Spergel, D.N. and Turok, N.G. 1992. "Textures and Cosmic Structures" in Scientific American. Mar. '92. N.Y.

2. Weinberg, Steven. (1987) "Toward the Final Laws of Physics" in Elementary Particles and the Laws of Physics. N.Y.: Cambridge University Press.

3. Weinberg, Steven (1992) Dreams of A Final Theory. N.Y.: Random House.

Chapter Thirteen

1. Clark, Ronald W. (1971) Article titled "The Revolution in Science" appearing in The Times, London, Nov. 7, 1919. (P. 297).

2. Rein, Glen. (1988) "Psychoenergetic Mechanism for Healing with Subtle Energies". Paper presented at the International Psychotronics Association conference at West Georgia College, Georgia.

3. Scott, Alwyn C. "The Solitary Wave:An Enduring Pulse First Seen in Water May Convey Energy in the Cell". The Sciences. Mar./Apr. 1990. N.Y.Academy of Sciences.

4. Scott, Alwyn C. (1990) ibid. P. 28-34.

5. Barrow, John D. (1988) <u>The World Within the World.</u> N.Y.: Oxford Press.

Chapter Fifteen

1. Pais, Abraham. (1991) <u>Niels Bohr's Times</u>. Oxford: Clarendon. P. 431.

2. Miller, Daniel. "Dissociation In Medical Practice". <u>Social Distress and Homelessness</u>. Fall, 1993 (to be issued).